Recovery and Stress in Sport

Balancing training, stress, and recovery is essential for achieving optimal performance. The performance of professional athletes can be severely compromised by overtraining, prolonged periods of competition, or even life events outside their sporting lives.

The current recovery-stress state depends on preceding stress and recovery activities, but through simultaneous assessment of stress and recovery, a differentiated picture can be provided. This manual includes two measurement instruments to gauge individual recovery, enabling both athletes and coaches to better understand the often-unconscious processes that impinge upon peak performance, and to monitor the physical, mental, emotional, and overall recovery-stress state before and after training. The *Acute Recovery and Stress Scale* (ARSS) and the *Short Recovery and Stress Scale* (SRSS) are instruments that systematically enlighten the recovery-stress states of athletes. Through utilization of the ARSS and the SRSS, athletes and coaches can better understand the importance of daily activities, including how they can relate to stress/recovery and the direct impact on athletic performance.

In addition to the instruments themselves, both of which are simple and easy to use, the manual also discusses their development, their basis in theory, and case studies showcasing their usage. The ARSS and the SRSS provide important information regarding the current recovery-stress state during the process of training, and are essential tools for coaches, sport psychologists, and athletes alike.

Michael Kellmann is Head of the Sport Psychology Unit, Faculty of Sport Science, Ruhr University Bochum, Germany and Honorary Professor at the School of Human Movement and Nutrition Sciences, The University of Queensland, Australia.

Sarah Kölling is a researcher and lecturer at the Sport Psychology Unit, Faculty of Sport Science, Ruhr University Bochum, Germany. While creating this manual, she also held a post-doc position at Stellenbosch University, South Africa.

Recovery and Stress in Sport
A Manual for Testing and Assessment

Michael Kellmann and Sarah Kölling

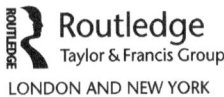

LONDON AND NEW YORK

First published 2019
by Routledge
2 Park Square, Milton Park, Abingdon, Oxon OX14 4RN

and by Routledge
52 Vanderbilt Avenue, New York, NY 10017

Routledge is an imprint of the Taylor & Francis Group, an informa business

© 2019 Michael Kellmann and Sarah Kölling

The right of Michael Kellmann and Sarah Kölling to be identified as authors of this work has been asserted by them in accordance with sections 77 and 78 of the Copyright, Designs and Patents Act 1988.

All rights reserved. No part of this book may be reprinted or reproduced or utilized in any form or by any electronic, mechanical, or other means, now known or hereafter invented, including photocopying and recording, or in any information storage or retrieval system, without permission in writing from the publishers.

Trademark notice: Product or corporate names may be trademarks or registered trademarks, and are used only for identification and explanation without intent to infringe.

British Library Cataloguing-in-Publication Data
A catalogue record for this book is available from the British Library

Library of Congress Cataloging-in-Publication Data
A catalog record for this book has been requested

ISBN: 978-1-138-38952-6 (hbk)
ISBN: 978-1-138-38953-3 (pbk)
ISBN: 978-0-429-42385-7 (ebk)

Typeset in Baskerville
by Apex CoVantage, LLC

Dedicated to all of the people who participated in the development of the *Acute Recovery and Stress Scale* as well as the *Short Recovery and Stress Scale*.

Contents

*User information for the Acute Recovery and Stress Scale and the Short Recovery
and Stress Scale*   x
Preface   xi
Acknowledgments   xii

1 Overview   1

2 Theory   2
Recovery and stress 2
Assessing recovery and stress in sport 4

3 Test development   6
Development of the German ARSS 6
   Phase I: preparatory phase 6
   Phase II: exploratory model development 6
   Phase III: confirmatory model verification 7
   Phase IV: confirmatory model verification with target group 8
Development of the German SRSS 8
Development of the English ARSS and SRSS 8
   Phase I 8
   Phase II 9
Validation of the German ARSS and SRSS, and the English ARSS and SRSS 9
Overview of samples and studies 11
   Sample GS1 11
   Sample GS2 11
   Sample GS3 11
   Sample GS4 11
   Sample GS5 13
   Sample ES1 13
   Sample ES2 14
Methods of analysis 14

4 The *Acute Recovery and Stress Scale*   16
Scope and application 16
   Sport-scientific practice 16
   Sport-scientific research 16
Instruction 16
Evaluation 17
Interpretation 17
   Recovery dimension 18
   Stress dimension 18

Reference values and scale statistics 19
Reliability 19
   Homogeneity 19
   Test-retest reliability 19
Construct validity 22
   Scale intercorrelations 22
   Factorial validity 24
Convergent and discriminant validity 28
   Correlations with actual mood state 28
   Sensitivity to change 31
   Performance parameters 34
   Physiological response 34
Summary of the ARSS 38

5   The *Short Recovery and Stress Scale*   39

Scope and application 39
   Sport-scientific practice 39
   Sport-scientific research 40
Instruction 40
Evaluation 40
Interpretation 40
   Short Recovery Scale 41
   Short Stress Scale 41
Reference values and item statistics 42
Reliability 42
   Homogeneity 42
   Test-retest reliability 43
Construct validity 44
   Item intercorrelations 44
Convergent and discriminant validity 45
   Correlations with actual mood state 45
   Sensitivity to change 49
   Performance parameters 53
   Physiological response 53
Summary of the SRSS 55

6   Comparison of the ARSS and the SRSS   56

Correlations between the ARSS and the SRSS 56
Comparison of construct validity 57
Comparison of sensitivity to change 58
Discussion of the ARSS and the SRSS 58
Recommendation for usage in practice 60
Conclusion 62

7   Case studies   63

References   67
Publications using the ARSS and/or the SRSS (Status: December 2018)   72

	Contents	ix
Appendix		74

   Appendix overview 74
   Appendix ARSS 75
   Appendix SRSS 87
   Appendix ARSS, scoring key and profile 89
   Appendix SRSS, scoring key and profile 95

About the authors   103
Index   104

User information for the *Acute Recovery and Stress Scale* and the *Short Recovery and Stress Scale*

Dear User,

Purchasing the *Acute Recovery and Stress Scale* (ARSS) and the *Short Recovery and Stress Scale* (SRSS) includes the right of unlimited duplication of the assessment tools. The only requirement is that you have purchased the original manual from Routledge.

If you use the ARSS/SRSS in your studies or in applied settings, the authors would appreciate feedback on your experience in working with these instruments. For further development of these instruments, we would be grateful if you could send us a copy of the original data set, a sample description, and information about the study or intervention approach used.

If you have further questions or comments, please contact:

Prof. Dr. Michael Kellmann and Dr. Sarah Kölling
Ruhr University Bochum, Faculty of Sport Science
Gesundheitscampus Nord 10, 44801 Bochum, Germany
E-Mail: Michael.Kellmann@rub.de; Sarah.Koelling@rub.de
www.spowiss.rub.de/sportpsych

Once purchased, you may use the ARSS/SRSS as research or monitoring tools for athletes during the training process. Athletes and coaches can modify the personal and training environment to optimize the training process and actively reduce the risk of overtraining. However, you should **not** use the ARSS/SRSS for selection purposes! Although there is a slight tendency to use the results of psychological assessments for selection decisions, this practice is unethical and may destroy the trusting relationship between coach and athlete. Furthermore, the consultation with a trained sport psychologist or counseling center, as well as medical advice is highly recommended if a serious long-lasting and unhealthy recovery-stress state is detected.

Please be aware that the authors hold the copyright for all languages. If you are interested in obtaining permission to translate and validate the ARSS and the SRSS into other languages, please contact the authors. In addition, you must have a background in psychometrics and you need to follow the translation procedure described by Vallerand (1989); see also 'Development of the English ARSS and SRSS' section in Chapter 3. Sometimes, researchers just translate an instrument without validation process and without receiving permission from the authors. Besides breaching the copyright, this may lead to difficulties in the development and interpretation. We are aware of cross-cultural differences which have an impact on the translation and as a result of variations of English around the world, we have included three different English language regions in our analysis. Furthermore, in some languages a direct translation of terms (without considering the content with the specific cultural background) leads to an unreliable translation. Therefore, the validation process needs to be solid and well documented.

Preface

This manual is the product of a research process, which took place within the framework of the joint project '*Optimization of Training and Competition: Management of Regeneration in Elite Sports* (REGman)' (ZMVI4–081901/12–20), funded by the German Federal Institute of Sport Science (BISp). This interdisciplinary project was part of the implementation of the research program for the Scientific Network System in High-Performance Sports[1] and was conducted by the Saarland University, Germany, under the lead of Tim Meyer (Saarland University, Germany, Sport Medicine), Alexander Ferrauti (Ruhr University Bochum, Germany, Training & Exercise Science), Mark Pfeiffer (Johannes Gutenberg University of Mainz, Germany, Training & Exercise Science), and Michael Kellmann (Ruhr University Bochum, Germany, Sport Psychology). Results and recommendations were published in a special brochure by the BISp (Meyer, Ferrauti, Kellmann, & Pfeiffer, 2016).

As one result of the project, a psychometric scale to assess acute recovery and stress in sport was developed. This scale served as an important basis for the main investigations, which were structured in three steps (Meyer et al., 2016): development of methods (step 1), intervention and field studies (step 2), and transfer of results (step 3). The development phase generated two psychometric instruments, which were successfully used in the REGman project[2] and are now established diagnostic instruments in German high-performance sport.

This manual describes the *Acute Recovery and Stress Scale* (ARSS) and the *Short Recovery and Stress Scale* (SRSS), which was derived from the ARSS in a tiered development process. Since the ARSS and the SRSS are two independent instruments, the questionnaires are described in separate chapters. Subsequently, there are repetitions for the sake of completeness.

When developed test instruments are translated into another language, the validation process is often perceived as shortened and less detailed than the original version. Consequently, this may impact the quality of the test instruments. However, since the structure of our instruments and items has already been developed in the original version, the translated version has a better starting point and is not inferior to the original version. Variations in reliability and validity may also be due to cultural differences and a slightly different understanding of the language. Due to variations of English around the world, some differences in interpretation of Australia/New Zealand, British, and North American English naturally occur. This became evident during the translation of the adjectives used in the ARSS/SRSS into English, as well as in the following back-to-back translation from experts from the three regions (Australia/New Zealand, United Kingdom, USA/Canada).

The German versions of the ARSS and the SRSS were published as a manual in 2016 that contains various validation studies (Kellmann, Kölling, & Hitzschke, 2016). Because of the current shortage of English validation studies of the final translated versions, the German studies are listed and described in this manual, as well. In the manual, we only use the English terms ARSS and SRSS. For clarification, when referring to the English versions, the ARSS and SRSS are the corresponding labels. The German versions are labeled as German ARSS and German SRSS.

Acknowledgments

Large projects, such as the development of the *Acute Recovery and Stress Scale* and the *Short Recovery and Stress Scale*, can only be realized with the unremitting effort of creative and motivated people. Our special thanks go to the REGman team consisting of Tim Meyer, Alexander Ferrauti, Mark Pfeiffer, Thimo Wiewelhove, Christian Raeder, Christian Rasche, Fabian Loch, Brit Hitzschke, Maximilian Pelka, and Annika Hof zum Berge, as well as to the BISp for funding the REGman project.

Special thanks go to Anna Schauerte, Denise Tautenhahn, and Brent Raiteri for supporting the translation and proofreading, Anu Nässi for performing the first validation study of the English ARSS, Paul Schaffran for running special analyses, Annika Hof zum Berge for creating the figures, and Asja Kiel for providing and checking tables.

Without the support of numerous people, the data collection process could not have been accomplished. Therefore, we would like to thank all of the anonymous athletes for contributing their time in the validation process and Richard Akenhead, Renee Appaneal, Louise Assioun, Jon Bartlett, Caleb Bazyler, Sophie Broome, Alan Bullock, Sarah Cheney, Justin Cordy, Aaron Coutts, Glenn Cundari, Bobby Davies, Craig Duncan, Mikah Van Gogh, Andrew Govus, Shona Halson, Tandy Haughey, Andrew Hawkins, Annika Hof zum Berge, Jonas Hummels, Vince Kelly, Emily Kraus, Simon Loftus, Cliff Mallet, Mollie Martin, Lara Meyer, Skate Miller, Pablo Nolte, Tom Patrick, Kirsten Peterson, Jonah Oliver, Michael O'Keeffe, Brent Raiteri, Georgia Ridler, Anna Schauerte, Robert Southall-Edwards, Billy Sperlich, Michael Stollberg, Michael Stone, Paul Turk, Lee Wallace, Mark Watsford, Simon Wheatley, and Ranel Venter for their support during athlete recruitment and data collection.

Special thanks to Ben Raysmith and Mick Drew from the Australian Institute of Sport and to Adam Bibbey from Oxford Brookes University in England for their various efforts recruiting athletes.

Notes

1 Wissenschaftliches Verbundsystem im Leistungssport
2 Publications of the REGman project are displayed at www.regman.org/publikationen

1 Overview

Application areas

The *Acute Recovery and Stress Scale* (ARSS) and *Short Recovery and Stress Scale* (SRSS) assess the current recovery-stress state of an athlete at an emotional, mental, physical, and overall level. They are developed for the use on active athletes aged 16 years and older. The SRSS is more economical (e.g., less time-consuming) and especially useful for high-frequency measurements (e.g., in the daily monitoring of training). The ARSS is better suited for deriving detailed information, which is useful for detecting smaller variations in an athlete's emotional or mental state.

The questionnaires

The questionnaires are standardized self-assessment procedures and include the scales/items *Physical Performance Capability*, *Mental Performance Capability*, *Emotional Balance*, and *Overall Recovery* in the dimension of *Recovery*; and *Muscular Stress*, *Lack of Activation*, *Negative Emotional State*, and *Overall Stress* in the dimension of *Stress*. The ARSS was constructed based on an expert survey, Exploratory and Confirmatory Factor Analyses, and consists of 32 adjectives. The scales are generated by calculating the mean value of those adjectives with four adjectives for each scale. The SRSS was derived from the eight scales of the ARSS which were then grouped into the *Short Recovery Scale* and the *Short Stress Scale* and consist of four items each. As descriptors, the adjectives from the ARSS are listed underneath the SRSS items for a better understanding only. In both questionnaires, the level of agreement is determined by a seven-point Likert scale ('0' = *does not apply at all* to '6' = *fully applies*).

Reliability

The internal consistency (Cronbach's α) for the ARSS ranges between $\alpha = .77$ and $\alpha = .88$ and for the SRSS between $\alpha = .78$ and $\alpha = .84$.

Validity

The factorial validity of the exploratory model was confirmed by using factor analyses. The construct validity is supported by theory-conform relationships with the established methods of the Recovery-Stress Questionnaire for Athletes (Kellmann & Kallus, 2001, 2016), Profile of Mood States (McNair, Lorr, & Droppleman, 1992) and the visual analogue scale to assess Delayed-Onset Muscle Soreness (Ohnhaus & Adler, 1975) in sport-specific stress and rest situations. The sensitivity to change could also be verified for both questionnaires in the training monitoring of different sports.

Duration

The ARSS takes between 4 and 5 minutes to complete (depending on the familiarity with the questionnaire). Completion of the SRSS takes between 40 and 60 seconds.

2 Theory

The balance between recovery and stress and between training and rest is of high importance in the daily routine of competitive athletes, and is a substantial component for optimal competition preparation (Hausswirth & Mujika, 2013; Kellmann & Beckmann, 2018a). Fast and effective regeneration and recovery have become important due to the increased frequency of competition, which is related to social and media pressures and the constant pursuit for performance improvement. The greater demand on athletes is supported by literature findings of inadequate recovery phases and overload symptoms in athletes from different sport disciplines (Dupont et al., 2010; Ekstrand, Walden, & Hagglund, 2004; Main & Landers, 2012; Meyer, 2010). Increased training stimuli for a long period combined with insufficient recovery can lead to a performance stagnation or decrease and may even involve a chronic maladaptation. This is known as overtraining syndrome (Meeusen et al., 2013; Meeusen & De Pauw, 2018). Progressive fatigue and underperformance can be the result of a long-term underrecovery (Halson, 2014; Kellmann & Beckmann, 2018a). However, the difficulty is to determine the exact point when conventional training turns from overreaching into non-functional overreaching.

Recovery and stress

Since the terms load and stress differ between scientific disciplines, it is necessary to define them.[1] *Load* defines the objectively quantifiable variables or factors that externally affect a person. Load is reflected in the subjective results and in the person's perception of *stress* (Rohmert & Rutenfranz, 1975). To give an example from sports, different individuals *respond* differently (subjective stress; e.g., dependent on the training condition or the current state on the day) to an external *load* of 100 kg in bench press (objective **load**). Also, the same individual may respond differently to the same external load because of changes in their current physiological, emotional, and mental states. Therefore, the assessment of the mediating psychological processes associated with various perceptions (e.g., perceptions of load/effort/discomfort) are of great importance (Jerusalem, 1990; Lazarus, 1991). Athletes with the same performance level may react in different ways to an identical stimulus and show different stress states (Raglin, 1993). The same external absolute training load could lead to the desired training adaptions in one athlete, but chronic maladaptations in another athlete (O'Toole, 1998), or even the same athlete under different stress and recovery states. Therefore, there is a need to assess the emotional and mental states of an athlete and potential regeneration/recovery strategies to help them adapt to stress.

Kellmann, Bertollo, et al. (2018) recently defined the terms that are related to recovery in a consensus statement.

> Recovery is regarded as a multifaceted (e.g., physiological, psychological) restorative process relative to time. In case an individual's recovery status (i.e., his or her biopsychosocial balance) is disturbed by external or internal factors, fatigue as a condition of augmented tiredness due to physical and mental effort develops. Fatigue can be compensated with recovery, that is, the organismic allostatic balance is regained by reestablishing the invested resources on a physiological and psychological level.
>
> (Kellmann, Bertollo, et al., 2018, p. 240)

Physiologically, recovery is mainly referred to as **regeneration** in sport and exercise contexts (Kellmann, Bertollo, et al., 2018). Ideally, regeneration follows physical fatigue that has been induced by training or competition. Nédélec et al. (2012) mentioned cold water immersion (CWI), nutrition/diet, and sleep as frequently used and scientifically evaluated regeneration methods. On a psychological level, cognitive coping strategies, resource activation, and psychological relaxation techniques (e.g., breathing, progressive muscle relaxation, systematic application of napping) help to reduce mental fatigue (Kellmann & Beckmann, 2018b; Kellmann, Pelka, & Beckmann, 2018; Pelka & Kellmann, 2017).

A continuous physiological or psychological imbalance due to inadequate recovery and excessive demands can be the result of insufficient systematic and individualized recovery, which can further lead to a cascade of deleterious conditions. The first precursor of an overtraining syndrome can be a state of continuous underrecovery which has been identified as underrecovery syndrome (Kellmann, Bertollo, et al., 2018). This **underrecovery syndrome** is the consequence of an imbalance between daily life demands and recovery, and depicts the reaction to general stress (e.g., family, media) as a broader condition of insufficient recovery. Meeusen et al. (2013), on the other hand, define **non-functional overreaching** (NFO) as a more training-specific concept that results in negative psychological and hormonal alterations and decreased performance. Continuous underrecovery and NFO often serve as precursors to overtraining syndrome. An accumulation of insufficient recovery from daily life demands, in combination with a long-term NFO in training and competition, will inevitably lead to the **overtraining syndrome**. Despite a considerable overlap in symptoms between underrecovery and overtraining (e.g., fatigue, exhaustion), physical symptoms of an overtrained state include continuous muscle soreness, pain sensations, or clinical and/or endocrinological disturbances. The earlier potential intervention strategies are applied, the shorter the recovery period from overtraining will be. Compensation for underrecovery can be the systematic application of recovery strategies and rest periods, while recovering from overtraining requires a continuous restoration. This can only be achieved through long rest periods that might last from weeks to months. **Recovery** serves as the umbrella term, which can then be further characterized by different forms of recovery, such as regeneration or psychological recovery strategies. These strategies should be applied in a structured manner and they should be tailored to the individual needs of the athlete.

It is certain that in sport and training science, the type of stimulus and the type of recovery interact with each other, depending on the respective activity (Kellmann, Bertollo, et al., 2018). A stimulus can, therefore, either lead to overload or, in combination with sufficient recovery, it can contribute to a training effect and an increased resilience to the training stimulus. Top athletic performance cannot only be accomplished through optimal training intensity and volume, but also through the compliance and facilitation of sufficient rest and recovery phases between training sessions (Hoffman, Epstein, Yarom, Zigel, & Einbinder, 1999). Chronic negative consequences in the mental and physical domain, for example as an overtraining syndrome, can be the result of neglected recovery (Kellmann, Bertollo, et al., 2018). Therefore, it is important to recognize an imbalance between the recovery-stress state as early as possible to avoid an unplanned reduction in performance (Brink, Visscher, Coutts, & Lemmink, 2012; Kellmann & Beckmann, 2018a). Standardized diagnostic methods can identify signs of overtraining with the help of the current biopsychosocial stress state to individually adapt the training regulation (Meeusen et al., 2013). Moreover, psychometric methods can support interdisciplinary cooperation between the coaches, medical team, and sport-psychological staff (Kellmann, Bertollo, et al., 2018). According to Hooper, Mackinnon, Howard, and Gordon (1995), the difficulty with physiological markers lies in distinguishing abnormal changes from normal reactions that result from intensive training stimuli. Often, overtraining syndromes are more effectively revealed with the help of psychological parameters than with objective tests (Kenttä & Hassmén, 1998; Raglin & Wilson, 2000; Saw, Main, & Gastin, 2016; Saw, Kellmann, Main, & Gastin, 2017).

Psychometric scales may well represent the most successful instrument in scientific studies to show recovery and stress (Heidari et al., 2019; Heidari, Kölling, Pelka, & Kellmann, 2018; Kellmann, Bertollo, et al., 2018; Meeusen et al., 2013; Nässi, Ferrauti, Meyer, Pfeiffer, & Kellmann, 2017b; Saw et al., 2016). One reason for this superiority could be assumed in the underlying global approach, as the gathered items assess several recovery and stress levels at the same time. The mental state, for instance, is constituted from different physical, mental, and emotional inputs that are processed by the central nervous system and hence influence the perception of the recovery-stress state, as well as the need for regeneration. By using psychometric methods, the individual biopsychosocial recovery-stress state can be measured economically and effectively and with as little impact as possible. In addition, performance control and training prescription can be supported (Meeusen et al., 2013). With regard to the monitoring of larger groups, using psychometric tools bears advantages due to the economy of implementation and the objectivity of evaluation (Kellmann & Beckmann, 2003). Furthermore, the recording of the athlete's subjective perspective is crucial for an early identification of fatigue and stress signals (Meeusen et al., 2013; Meeusen & De Pauw,

2018). Constant monitoring is especially relevant, as athletes react differently and adapt individually to training stimuli (Coutts, Crowcroft, & Kempton, 2018; Hecksteden et al., 2017). It should be considered, though, that psychometric methods are generally transparent and are therefore easy to manipulate, as well. Hence, the use of the data and the benefit for an optimal training prescription must be explained to the athletes (Kellmann & Beckmann, 2003).

Assessing recovery and stress in sport

The following subjective measurements are mostly used in sport-scientific research and practice: Borg's Rating of Perceived Exhaustion (Borg, 1998), Delayed-Onset Muscle Soreness (Ohnhaus & Adler, 1975), Profile of Mood States (McNair, Lorr, & Droppleman, 1992) and Recovery-Stress Questionnaire for Athletes (Kellmann & Kallus, 2001, 2016).

Borg's Rating of Perceived Exhaustion (RPE; Borg, 1998) is a one-dimensional scale. The original version with a scale from 6 to 20 (*very, very easy* to *very, very hard*) measures the training intensity and the perceived exhaustion of an athlete at a certain time. Due to its shortness, the RPE has been used in many experimental studies (Noble & Robertson, 1996). Changes in the RPE scale in combination with blood lactate proved to be a reliable predictor for overtraining (Snyder, 1998; Snyder, Jeukendrup, Hesselink, Kuipers, & Foster, 1993). In a cohort study with more than 2,500 participants, the RPE turned out to be a convenient and valid instrument for emphasizing the training intensity independently from gender, age, and type of the implemented load (Scherr et al., 2013). Foster (1998) introduced a modification of the RPE (Session-RPE), which involves an athlete rating a whole training session with a global intensity. By multiplying the value (on a scale from 0 to 10) with the duration of the training session 30 minutes after completion, the individual training load can also be determined (Impellizzeri, Rampinini, Coutts, Sassi, & Marcora, 2004). However, a criticism of RPE scales is that the underlying reasons for changes in subjective effort across sessions for the same absolute training load remain unclear. Therefore, it is difficult to derive appropriate intervention measures based on the ratings alone (Mäetsu, Jürimäe, & Jürimäe, 2005). For example, athletes who were identified with overtraining syndrome showed only minor variation in RPE ratings (Urhausen & Kindermann, 2002). Kellmann (2002) has pointed out that by using a 'one-item scale', the multidimensional aspect of stress and recovery is neglected. Moreover, Kenttä and Hassmén (1998) argue that recovery, which they do not only characterize as the absence or reduction of stress, is completely disregarded.

In training and (sports-)medical or clinical settings, the visual analogue scale has been used to measure Delayed-Onset Muscle Soreness (DOMS; Ohnhaus & Adler, 1975). The athlete marks on a 10-cm line, ranging from *no pain* (left endpoint) to *extreme pain* (right endpoint), the appropriate position for his/her experienced pain intensity. The distance (in mm or cm) between the left endpoint and the respective mark represents the pain index. Consequently, the scale proves to be an economical and quickly implemented method, which is especially useful in experimental studies (Brown et al., 2017; Cleather & Guthrie, 2007; Nosaka, Newton, & Sacco, 2002; Page, Swan, & Patterson, 2017). Williamson and Hoggart (2005) observed a good sensitivity to change in pain perception and a high retest reliability. However, the level of DOMS is a one-dimensional construct as well, which is restricted to the muscular component of stress.

Another widely used instrument is the Profile of Mood States (POMS; McNair et al., 1992), which measures the current mood state of a person. It is a 65-item questionnaire consisting of five negative affect scales, namely *Tension, Depression, Anger, Fatigue*, and *Confusion*, and one positive affect scale of *Vigor*. A global score of *Total Mood Disturbance* can be calculated by subtracting the *Vigor* score from the sum of the scores of the five remaining scales. This instrument is typically administered with instructions to respond on the basis of feelings experienced in a specific time frame. Although the method was originally developed for the clinical-psychological context, it is a frequently used instrument in overtraining research and in sport-scientific practice (e.g., Bresciani et al., 2011; Raglin, Morgan, & O'Connor, 1991; Slivka, Hailes, Cuddy, & Ruby, 2010; Ten Haaf et al., 2017). For instance, a correlation between training volume and change of mood was visible insofar that an increased training load led to a deterioration of mood, while a training reduction led to an improvement of mood (Raglin, 1993). However, as this instrument is not a sport-specific tool, no explicit recommendations for performance control and training prescription/intervention can be derived from it (Kellmann, 2002). Moreover, the dimensions of the POMS do not cover the recovery aspect sufficiently (Mäetsu et al., 2005).

The presumably best-known instrument in the context of sport is the Recovery-Stress Questionnaire for Athletes (RESTQ-Sport; Kellmann & Kallus, 2001, 2016). With 76 items, the RESTQ-Sport-76 assesses potentially stressful events and their consequences on an athlete, along with the frequency of recovery-associated activities and their effects in the previous three days/nights. These items are summarized in 12 general and seven sport-specific scales, and provide the individual recovery-stress profile. The RESTQ-Sport helps to identify an imbalance in the recovery-stress state, which can be used as an early indicator for overtraining symptoms. The usefulness of the RESTQ-Sport has been shown in numerous studies regarding monitoring of training, as well as prevention of injury and overtraining (e.g., Bresciani et al., 2011; Brink et al., 2012; Coutts, Wallace, & Slattery, 2007; di Fronso, Nakamura, Bortoli, Robazza, & Bertollo, 2013; Hough, Corney, Kouris, & Gleeson, 2013; Laux, Krumm, Diers, & Flor, 2015; Meister, Faude, Amman, Schnittker, & Meyer, 2013; Otter, Brink, van der Does, & Lemmink, 2016; van der Does, Brink, Otter, Visscher, & Lemmink, 2017; for an overview, see Kellmann & Kallus, 2016). A prominent example of differences in the recovery potential of two athletes in their RESTQ-Sport profiles are two rowers participating in the Olympic Games. The rower with the more favorable profile finished the competition as a medalist, while the other rower came 13th (Kellmann & Günther, 2000). Furthermore, the RESTQ-Sport could differentiate between two groups: one which had a normal training volume, and the other which had an increased training intensity (Coutts et al., 2007). The recovery-stress state also correlates with performance parameters and biological markers, e.g., cortisol, testosterone, and creatine kinase (Auersperger et al., 2014; Bouget, Rouveix, Michaux, Pequignot, & Filaire, 2006; dos Santos, Kuczynski, Machado, Osiecki, & Stefanello, 2014; Garatachea et al., 2011; Skovgaard et al., 2014). Since the publication of a new edition of the RESTQ's manual in 2016, a reduced version with 36 items has also been made available. This version includes six general and six sport-specific scales (Kellmann & Kallus, 2016).

Applied assessment tools need to be specifically developed for athletes while still fulfilling the psychometric requirements. Economic measures already exist with the RPE and DOMS, and multidimensional methods can be found in the RESTQ-Sport and the POMS. However, no method that combines all three – multidimensionality, sport-specificity, and economy – has currently been developed. The continuous measuring of the recovery-stress state for three consecutive days and nights complicates its usage over short intervals (e.g., multiple measurements within a week) and it does not provide any information about the current or *acute* recovery-stress state. Consequently, there is no method that measures and presents the multidimensional *acute* recovery-stress state sport-specifically, economically, and in a way that is sensitive to change.

The development of the *Acute Recovery and Stress Scale* (ARSS) and the *Short Recovery and Stress Scale* (SRSS) closes this gap in research, and meets the sport-practical demands for a quick assessment that has theoretical underpinnings.

Note

1 The definitions are common in the field of work psychology. For more information about the distinction between strain, load, and stress, see Kallus (2016).

3 Test development

In the following sections, the implemented steps of the test development, which consisted of a construction and a validation phase, are outlined. To illustrate the process, these steps are summarized in Figure 3.1. The Appendix overview provides a summary of the original German items and the translated items, which were used in the different stages of the development of the ARSS. Hitzschke et al. (2015, 2016, 2017) and Kellmann et al. (2016) have already published the construction process and the first results from the German ARSS and the German SRSS in detail. In addition, the validity and sensitivity were verified in various laboratory studies (e.g., Hammes et al., 2016; Hitzschke et al., 2017; Julian et al., 2017; Pelka, Ferrauti, Meyer, Pfeiffer, & Kellmann, 2017; Pelka, Kölling, et al., 2017; Raeder et al., 2016; Schimpchen et al., 2017; Wiewelhove et al., 2015, 2016, 2018) and field studies (e.g., Collette, 2016; Collette, Kellmann, Ferrauti, Meyer, & Pfeiffer, 2018; Kölling et al., 2015, 2016; Pelka, Schneider, & Kellmann, 2018; Puta et al., 2018; Zinner et al., 2017).

Development of the German ARSS

The development of the German ARSS (Kellmann et al., 2016) was carried out in four sequential phases (see Figure 3.1), consisting of a preparatory phase, two preliminary studies with German samples (GS1 and GS2, see Table 3.1), and a main study with the German target group of elite athletes (GS3, see Figure 3.1).

Phase I: preparatory phase

The development of the questionnaire was based on the concept of a multidimensional approach (physiological, mental, and emotional) to describe recovery and stress of an athlete and on the assumption that recovery and stress are two independent constructs (Kellmann, 2010; Kenttä & Hassmén, 1998). In a first step, qualitative ($N = 18$) and quantitative expert interviews ($N = 20$) were conducted and evaluated based on Mayring's (2010) Qualitative Data Analysis. The results were used to create an item pool and the initial adjective list.

Phase II: exploratory model development

In study GS1, the adjective and the item list were simultaneously used on 257 sport students to see which format was the most sensitive. Moreover, participants did a survey to determine their preference towards the end of the study and, in addition, they completed the RESTQ-Sport-76, so that first indicators to construct validity could be derived. The vote as well as the statistical calculations showed a trend towards the use of adjectives, so this format was used in further development. Based on the results of an Exploratory Factor Analysis and Reliability Analyses and following Kenttä and Hassmén (1998) and Kellmann (2010), one model each for recovery and stress was developed and the adjective list was modified accordingly. A first selection by means of item difficulty and diffusion (selection criteria: $1.5 < M < 4.5$, and $SD > 1.20$) was made and following this, the reduced version was used to calculate an Exploratory Factor Analysis. As covariance relationships between the latent variables are presumed, a Principal Component Analysis with an Oblique Promax Rotation was carried out. The number of factors was determined by the Minimum Average Partial Test (O'Connor, 2000). Criteria for the allocation of the items to the factors were the factor loading, the quality of the interpretability of the content and the item variance clarification by their respective factors when having items with double loading (Fürntratt criterion: $a^2/h^2 > .5$; Fürntratt, 1969). With these factors, a Reliability Analysis was calculated once again by means of the selection criteria $r_{it} > .30$

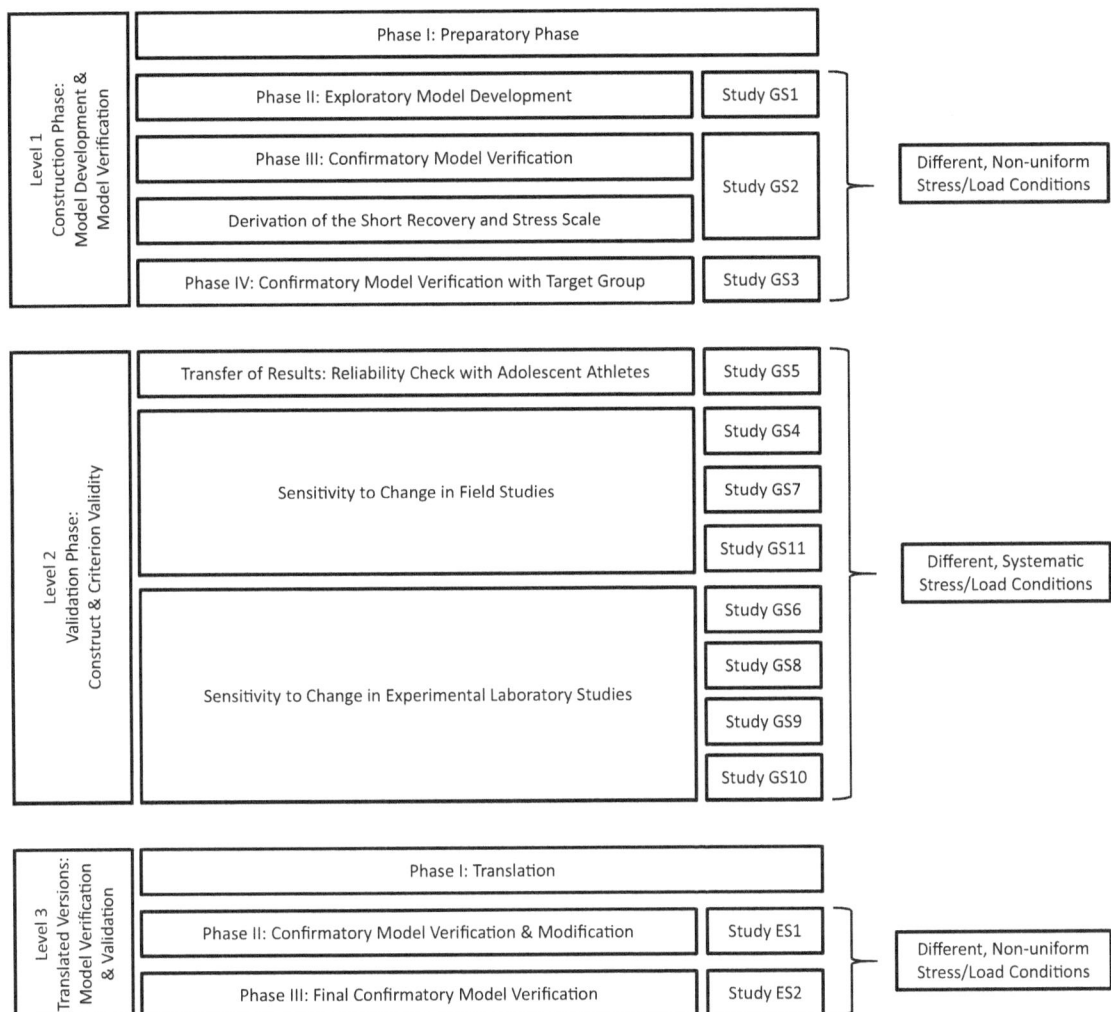

Figure 3.1 Stages of the test development and validation

and α > .70 (Lienert & Raatz, 1998). In addition, following first calculations of construct validity with the RESTQ-Sport-76, another item selection was implemented. The resulting adjective list after these steps was named *Acute Recovery and Stress Scale*. The aim was the development of several homogeneous scales with a small number of adjectives to realize a multidimensional and economical measurement. As a result of this development process, the scales *Physical Performance Capability*, *Mental Performance Capability*, *Emotional Balance* and *Overall Recovery* represent the *Recovery* dimension. The *Stress* dimension comprises the scales *Muscular Stress*, *Lack of Activation*, *Negative Emotional State*, and *Overall Stress*. The *Recovery* dimension, in particular, fulfills the current suggestion by Ten Haaf et al. (2017) to include the subjective mental and physical readiness to perform when monitoring fatigue.

Phase III: confirmatory model verification

Study GS2 included the ARSS, the RESTQ-Sport-76 and the DOMS, which were handed out to 429 performance-oriented female and male athletes.[1] The aim of the study was to verify the exploratory model of the ARSS with a Confirmatory Factor Analysis (CFA), to test the modifications that were made, to adjust the ARSS accordingly and to get the first information about the construct validity through the RESTQ-Sport-76 and the DOMS. An Exploratory Data Analysis was conducted first, followed by a Reliability Analysis and correlation calculations with the RESTQ-Sport-76 and the DOMS. Subsequently, a CFA was implemented. In preparation, the scales were checked for collinearity (correlations < .85), the existence of a multivariate normal distribution (Mardia's test) and the linearity of the correlations. The Maximum-Likelihood Estimation method was used, which is stable against violations of the Normal Distribution Assumption when having a kurtosis < 7, a skew < 2 and a sample size > 100 (see McDonald & Ho, 2002; West, Finch, & Curran, 1995). Bühner (2011) advised using the Maximum-Likelihood Estimation as a standard method. As recommended by Beauducel and Wittmann (2005), the following fit indices were used to evaluate the model adjustment: χ^2 and the corresponding p-value, *Comparative Fit Index* (CFI), *Root Mean Square Error of Approximation* (RMSEA), *Standardized Root Mean Residual* (SRMR), *Lower Limit of the 90%-Confidence Interval* (LO90), and *Upper Limit of the 90%-Confidence Interval* (HI90). The fit indices were assessed with the help of the threshold values (RMSEA ≤ .08, SRMR ≤ .10, CFI ≥ .90) summarized by Weiber and Mühlhaus (2010) and based on Browne and Cudeck (1993), Hu and Bentler (1999), and Homburg and Giering (1996).

Phase IV: confirmatory model verification with target group

The main study (GS3) was conducted to validate the results from the first two studies consisting of sport students and performance-oriented athletes with regard to elite sports ($N = 574$). The aim was to prove the transferability and stability of the model's structure by replicating the model and the construct validity correlations. Again, the ARSS, the DOMS, and the RESTQ-Sport-76 were used in the data collection. As in study GS2, a CFA (using the same criteria mentioned above) followed an Exploratory Data Analysis and a Reliability Analysis.

Development of the German SRSS

Regarding the content and the statistics, the SRSS was derived from the ARSS to create a stringent model-theoretical depiction and to support a mutual interpretation with the ARSS in the long run. Hence, the items of the SRSS reproduce the factor structure of the ARSS upon which the shorter version is based. With the help of the confirmatory calculations, a better model fit could be obtained for the ARSS when calculating the models for recovery and stress separately compared to a combined model calculation (Hitzschke et al., 2016). On this basis, the two dimensions *Recovery* and *Stress* were created and the SRSS was then subdivided into a *Short Recovery Scale* and a *Short Stress Scale*. The *Short Recovery Scale* consists of the items *Physical Performance Capability*, *Mental Performance Capability*, *Emotional Balance*, and *Overall Recovery*. The *Short Stress Scale* comprises the items *Muscular Stress*, *Lack of Activation*, *Negative Emotional State*, and *Overall Stress*. The items of the SRSS are named after the factors of the two confirmatory models or rather after the scales that were derived from the ARSS. Hence, the same terms are used. Through the development of the SRSS based on the derivation of items from the factor structure of the ARSS, an adaption to the ARSS and a joint application and interpretation should be facilitated in the long term. The development of the SRSS was highlighted by Horvath and Röthlin (2018) as one approach on how to shorten questionnaires in the applied sport psychology setting to improve their usability.

Development of the English ARSS and SRSS

Phase I

In phase I of the development, the English versions of the ARSS and the SRSS were translated with a parallel back-to back translation (Vallerand, 1989) by experts in the field of sport psychology (Figure 3.1). These experts, including staff members of the Faculty of Sport Science at the Ruhr University Bochum (Germany) and three expert coaches, translated the items of the questionnaires individually and met afterwards to discuss the translations and the items. Several bilingual experts with different cultural backgrounds (i.e., Australian, British, and North American) offered multiple back translations. Regardless of the form of English that was used, there was agreement for 87% of the items. The remaining 13% were seen ambiguously in their wording and meaning. The final call on the items was made by colleagues from Australia, who identified and modified items for the intended understanding in the Australian context.

On the basis of the back-to-back translation, it was decided to include additional items for three scales and to establish the final item wording based on values of Cronbach's α and CFA. Afterwards, a total of 36 items were sent to two additional experts in the field of sport science. Two items were modified after the experts' feedback to ensure a better understanding. The initial English versions of the ARSS and SRSS, which included 36 adjectives, were reduced to 32 items for the final version of the ARSS. The original item order of the German version was used, as statistical measures to avoid sequence effects had been applied during the initial questionnaire development. Four additional items were listed at the end of the ARSS and as descriptors of the corresponding SRSS items.

The survey links were distributed by the authors via sport institutions or clubs and sport associations. Each participant received information about the design and content of the study. The voluntary nature of participation was highlighted and informed consent was obtained. In addition to answering the ARSS, SRSS, and RESTQ-Sport-76 or POMS, the participants provided sociodemographic information. The procedures were in accordance with the Declaration of Helsinki and were approved by the local ethics committee.

Phase II

The data collection in phase II was conducted to confirm the theoretical model using CFA and to calculate Cronbach's α for the scales. As a possible backup, two more items were added to the scale *Emotional Balance* of the ARSS version as used in phase I. As a result, the SRSS item *Emotional Balance* contained six items as descriptors.

Again, the survey links were distributed online by the authors via sport institutions or clubs and sport associations. To avoid a language bias from Australian, British, or North American English, there was an intention to collect data from more than 300 participants in each language group. This sample was necessary for the CFA and to confirm that the model could be applied in all language regions. To our knowledge, this was the first time in sport psychology and sport science a psychometric instrument was simultaneously developed and validated for different language regions.

Prior to taking the survey, each participant received information about the design and the content of the study. The voluntary nature of participation was highlighted, and the participants signed an informed consent form. In addition to answering the ARSS, SRSS, and RESTQ-Sport-76 or POMS, the participants provided sociodemographic information. The procedures were authorized by the local ethics committee and conducted in accordance with the Declaration of Helsinki.

Validation of the German ARSS and SRSS, and the English ARSS and SRSS

The validation studies (GS4–GS12, summarized in Table 3.1) were conducted to verify the assumption that the model of acute recovery and stress, which was created under rest or uncontrolled stress conditions, could be replicated in stress situations, as well as to prove the model's sensitivity to change and its construct validity with different target populations.

The first validation study (GS4) was carried out as a field study and aimed at proving the ARSS's and SRSS's sensitivity to change in the presentation of recovery and stress processes during different stress situations (Hitzschke et al., 2015; Kölling et al., 2015). In addition, the reliability of the model of recovery and stress, as well as the construct validity with the RESTQ-Sport-76 was tested under stress conditions. The setting of a five-day field hockey training camp of the German female U21 national team was used to perform repeated and controlled field measurements with the target population.

Another validation study was conducted with adolescent male and female handball players to test the psychometric properties on a younger sample (GS5). To make sure the adolescents replied truthfully to the items, the option *I don't understand* was added. The validity of the ARSS was also tested in a laboratory study with cyclists in a microcycle with an intensive and high training volume (study GS6, Hammes et al., 2016). In addition, the suitability of the ARSS was examined for an extensive application for long-term monitoring in swimming by means of individual case and time-series analyses (study GS7, Collette, 2016; Collette et al., 2018).

The validity of the SRSS was confirmed by three laboratory studies. Study GS8 focused on the influence of an intensive strength training on fatigue parameters (Raeder et al., 2016), while study GS10 focused on the effect of different psychological recovery strategies (Pelka, Kölling, et al., 2017). Wiewelhove et al. (2016) investigated the effectiveness of active and passive recovery in a high-intensity interval training with young elite tennis players (study GS9). Furthermore, a four-week field study with the U19 national team of the German Rowing Association ($N = 55$) was implemented during their training camp with a focus on the relation with sleep parameters with the German SRSS (study GS11, Kölling et al., 2016).

Table 3.1 German research samples used to test validity and reliability of the ARSS and SRSS

Sample	N	Age M ± SD	Gender ♂	Gender ♀	Instruments	Times	Sport/Athletes	Publication
GS1	257	22.8 ± 3.1	190	67	Adjectives/sentences (ARSS), RESTQ-Sport	1	Sport science students	Hitzschke et al., 2016
GS2	429	25.3 ± 7.0	210	219	ARSS, SRSS, RESTQ-Sport, DOMS	1	Performance-oriented athletes	Hitzschke et al., 2016
GS3	574	21.0 ± 6.8	280	294	ARSS, SRSS, RESTQ-Sport, DOMS	1	Cadre athletes (national teams)	Hitzschke et al., 2015
GS4	25	19.1 ± 0.8	–	25	ARSS, SRSS, RESTQ-Sport, DOMS	5 days, frequently during the days	Field hockey, U21 national team	Hitzschke et al., 2015; Kölling et al., 2015 unpublished
GS5	239	15.2 ± 0.7	120	119	ARSS, SRSS	4 days, 2 times daily	Handball, developing athletes	Hammes et al., 2016
GS6	23	28.8 ± 7.6	23	–	ARSS	11 days, morning	Cyclists and triathletes	Collette, 2016
GS7	9	19.3 ± 3.1	–	9	ARSS, SRSS	48–152 days, morning	Swimming, national competing athletes	Raeder et al., 2016
GS8	23	24.8 ± 2.0	14	9	SRSS	11 days, mornings	Power lifters	Wiewelhove et al., 2016
GS9	8	15.1 ± 1.4	8	–	SRSS	2 (5 days apart)	Tennis, developing athletes	
GS10	27	25.2 ± 1.1	19	8	SRSS	1 day, 4 times daily	Sport science students	Pelka, Kölling, et al., 2017
GS11	55	17.7 ± 0.6	30	25	SRSS, sleep protocol	26 days, morning	Rowing, U19 national team	Kölling et al., 2016
GS12	25	17.5 ± 0.5	25	–	SRSS	12 weeks, 2 times weekly	Football, U19 Bundesliga team	Pelka et al., 2018

Note. ARSS = Acute Recovery and Stress Scale; SRSS = Short Recovery and Stress Scale; RESTQ-Sport = Recovery-Stress Questionnaire for Athletes; DOMS = Delayed-Onset Muscle Soreness; GS = German sample; Times = Frequency of measurements

The publication by Nässi et al. (2017a) describes the translation process and presents the first data of the English versions of the ARSS and SRSS (sample ES1, summarized in Table 3.2). Sample ES2 consists of various subsamples as described in the next chapter.

Overview of samples and studies

The following chapter describes the samples and the design of the construction and validation studies that were listed in Table 3.1 (samples GS1–GS5). Further studies that used the ARSS and/or SRSS will be described in detail in the psychometric properties sections in the respective chapters. When looking at the recruitment of participants, it should be considered that a tiered approach to the target population (i.e., elite athletes) was used in the construction phase for reasons of sample economy. Only in study GS3 did the sample consist of female and male competitive athletes. The age structure in the types of sport analyzed in samples GS2 and GS3 differed depending on the sport (e.g., gymnastics vs. golf). As a result, there was a broad age range in the samples. As the samples included older female and male athletes, a selection was made according to the indicated number of training hours per week (>8 hours) instead of using age as a selection criterion.

Sample GS1

The first paper-pencil version of the questionnaire consisted of an adjective and an item list. Sport students ($N = 257$) completed the German ARSS together with the RESTQ-Sport-76 under resting conditions in various uncontrolled situations (i.e., during a lecture, before and/or after training). The age distribution within the sample ranged from 18 to 44 years ($M = 22.8 \pm 3.1$ years). At the time of the survey, the students trained on average 10 ± 4.2 hours per week. Despite the small number of squad or national athletes and athletes who were active on a high competition level, 56% of the participants stated that they regularly participated in competitions.

Sample GS2

The sample consisted of 429 performance-oriented athletes who trained at least three times per week (training volume per week: 10.7 ± 4.4 hours). The age of the sample ranged from 16 to 56 years ($M = 25.3 \pm 7.0$ years). Altogether, the level of competition was higher than in study GS1 and more athletes belonged to a squad. Moreover, 92% confirmed their participation in competitions. Four percent of participants stated that they were part of a national team. The participants completed paper-pencil and online versions of the questionnaire.

Sample GS3

The 574 competitive female and male athletes from 15 to 62 years ($M = 21.0 \pm 6.8$ years) who participated in this study were recruited via Olympic Training Centers, cooperating sport associations, and through national coaches and coaches of the different federal states. The participant group were top-performing athletes who competed at a high level and belonged to a top team. The majority of athletes (63%) were part of a national team. At the time of the survey, athletes trained 14.9 ± 6.8 hours and participated in competitions regularly (97% of the participants). Participants were asked to fill in a paper-pencil or an online version of the questionnaire.

Sample GS4

Sample GS4 consisted of 25 female field hockey players of the German U21 national team. At the time of the investigation, the participants were 18–20 years old ($M = 19.1 \pm 0.8$ years). The study was conducted during a five-day training camp in preparation for the World Youth Championship. The paper-pencil questionnaires were completed on site. Due to different arrival and departure times and occasional absences of the athletes, the size of the sample varies slightly. Additions can be found in Kölling et al. (2015) for the ARSS evaluation and Hitzschke et al. (2015) for the SRSS analyses.

Figure 3.2 provides an overview of volume and content of the eight training blocks, the 13 points of measurement, measurement methods and the subjective assessment of the coach regarding the intensity of the individual training blocks. The coach assessed the training intensity on a seven-point Likert scale from '0' (*no intensity*) to '6' (*maximum intensity*).

Table 3.2 English research samples used to test validity and reliability of the ARSS and SRSS

Sample	N	Age M ± SD	Gender ♂	Gender ♀	Instruments# ARSS	Instruments# SRSS	Instruments# RESTQ-Sport	Instruments# POMS	Times	Sport/Athletes	Publication
ES1	267	25.2 ± 8.9	153	114	267	254	267	–	1	Elite/performance-oriented athletes	Nässi et al., 2017
ES2 (total)	1,039	24.8 ± 8.9	553	486	1,039	907	572	114	1	Elite/performance-oriented athletes	Kölling et al., submitted
ES2_ANZ	380	25.5 ± 9.8	213	167	380	375	239	61	1	Australian elite athletes	Kölling et al., submitted
ES2_UK	316	26.0 ± 9.8	158	158	316	304	126	42	1	British elite/performance-oriented athletes	Kölling et al., submitted
ES2_NA*	300	23.0 ± 6.6	165	135	300	186	165	11	1	US, Canadian elite/performance-oriented athletes	Kölling et al., submitted
ES2_NA_I	191	24.8 ± 7.5	117	74	191	184	165	11	1	US, Canadian elite/performance-oriented athletes	Kölling et al., submitted
ES2_NA_II	109	19.8 ± 1.2	48	61	109	–	–	–	7	US college athletes	Cheney et al., submitted
ES2_SA	43	23.0 ± 4.5	17	26	43	42	42	–	1	South African performance-oriented athletes	unpublished

Note: ARSS = *Acute Recovery and Stress Scale*; SRSS = *Short Recovery and Stress Scale*; RESTQ-Sport = Recovery-Stress Questionnaire for Athletes; POMS = Profile of Mood States; ES = English sample; ANZ = Australia/New Zealand; UK = United Kingdom; NA = North America; SA = South-Africa; Times = Frequency of measurements

* = North American sample consists of the subsamples ES2_NA_I (online data collection) and ES2_NA_II (Bachelor thesis with repeated measurements where the numbers over time vary slightly)

= The number of participants in the analysis of the ARSS and SRSS varies marginally and is dependent on complete data sets

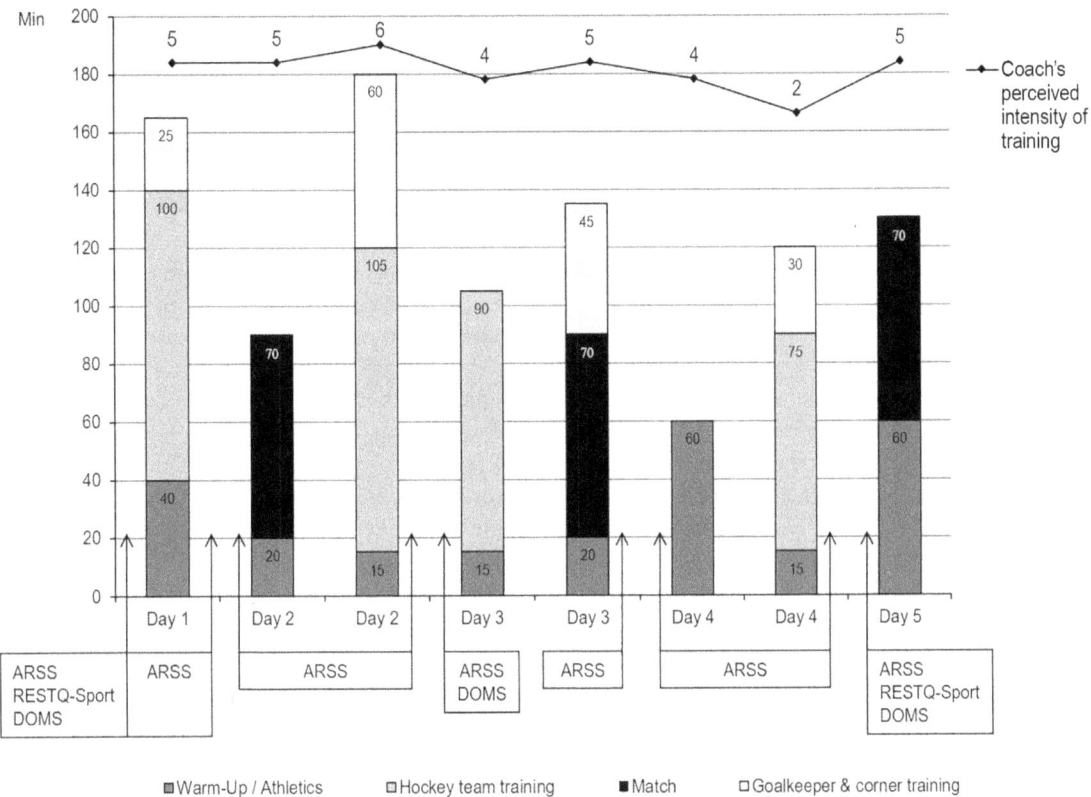

Figure 3.2 Procedure and schedule of the study GS4

Note: ARSS = *Acute Recovery and Stress Scale*; RESTQ-Sport = Recovery-Stress Questionnaire for Athletes; DOMS = Delayed-Onset Muscle Soreness

Source: reprinted, with permission, from Kölling et al., 2015, p. 532

During the training camp, athletes completed the German ARSS together with the German SRSS every morning and evening after their meals. In addition, athletes were asked to fill in the SRSS after lunch and on day 4 after the lunchbreak (Hitzschke et al., 2015). These separate SRSS measurements were made to check the sensitivity to change of the SRSS when completed within short time intervals, without overly disturbing the training process. Moreover, the single measurements were conducted to check cumulative effects of the training. The last data collection took place after breakfast on day 5. The RESTQ-Sport-76 was completed at the beginning and end of the training camp, and the DOMS was used at the beginning, middle, and end of the camp.

Sample GS5

The aim of study GS5 was to check the psychometric properties of the German ARSS and the German SRSS on 119 female and 120 male adolescent handball players from 13 to 16 years ($M = 15.2 \pm 0.7$ years). Both questionnaires were completed every morning and evening of a four-day talent scouting training course. The first measurement was taken on the first evening of the course. The athletes and their parents were informed in advance about the intervention and signed an informed consent form. They were assured that their responses would not influence the following talent assessment.

Sample ES1

Study ES1 aimed to evaluate the psychometric properties of the English ARSS and SRSS. The sample of the study consisted of 267 English-speaking athletes (114 females, 153 males) who independently completed online versions of the ARSS and SRSS questionnaires. On average, participants were 25.2 years old

($SD = 8.9$), with a range from 13 to 53 years, and trained 8.4 hours per week ($SD = 6.6$). Eighty-six percent of the sample regularly competed at a regional level or higher, while the remaining 14% were recreational athletes. The type of sport was relatively evenly distributed with 52% of the athletes participating in team ball sports and 48% engaging in an individual sport (e.g., athletics, triathlon, martial arts). The majority of the participants were from Australia (65%). The remaining athletes came from North America (21%), the United Kingdom (12%), and Ireland (2%). Of this sample, 95% ($n = 254$) also completed the SRSS.

Sample ES2

Study ES2 was conducted to confirm the model of the English ARSS and SRSS for different regions and to check for a potential language bias. For this purpose, the overall sample of ES2 was split into four sub-samples: ES2_ANZ (athletes from Australia and New Zealand), ES2_UK (athletes from the United Kingdom), ES2_NA (athletes from North America: USA, Canada), and ES2_SA (athletes from South Africa).

The overall sample of the study consisted of 1,039 English-speaking athletes (486 females, 553 males) who completed an online version of the ARSS and SRSS questionnaires. On average, participants were 24.8 years old ($SD = 8.9$) and trained 10.6 hours per week ($SD = 13.5$). The majority of the sample regularly competed on a regional level or higher (81.5%), 5% were collegiate athletes, and the remaining 13.5% were recreational athletes. The type of sport was relatively evenly distributed, with 53% of the athletes participating in team ball sports and 47% engaging in individual sports (e.g., athletics, triathlon, martial arts). The SRSS was also completed by 907 athletes from the sample (87%).

Of the 1,039 athletes who participated in the data assessment, 380 belonged to the subsample ES2_ANZ, 316 to the subsample ES2_UK, and 300 to the subsample ES2_NA. The latter consisted of the online survey and the study by Ms. Sarah Cheney (for details, see ahead). Forty-three athletes of the total sample ES2 were South African and belonged to the subsample ES2_SA (for details of the subsamples, see Table 3.2). Selected online links included the RESTQ-Sport-76 ($n = 569$) or the POMS ($n = 114$) for cross-validation.

Sample ES2_NA_II was collected in a Bachelor-Thesis by Ms. Sarah Cheney (Georgetown University, USA) in a study to test regeneration methods within a cross-over design (seven measurements). The measurements T1, T3, and T5 took place before training and are, therefore, considered to be rather similar compared to the other measurements that assessed the effect of the regeneration method. The ES2_NA_II subsample consisted of 109 performance-oriented US college athletes from cross country running, swimming, soccer, volleyball, lacrosse, American football, and field hockey (for details of the subsamples, see Table 3.2). The data of the first assessment were included into the ARSS analysis of homogeneity. Furthermore, test-retest correlations across time are displayed in Table 4.6.

It must be noted that the sample ES2 completed the revised English ARSS and SRSS versions (see phase I under the section 'Development of the English ARSS and SRSS') with two reserve items. While these reserve items (*stable* and *pleased*) were added at the end of the ARSS (items 33 and 34), they were also listed as descriptors for the SRSS item *Emotional Balance*.

Methods of analysis

Methods from Classical Test Theory as depicted in Lord and Novick (1968) were used to evaluate the psychometric quality of the different versions of the ARSS and SRSS. Correlations were computed as Spearman coefficients using the statistical software SPSS and other procedures are mentioned in the respective chapters. For validity analysis, Exploratory Factor Analyses were run for the scales by SPSS using the extraction of principal components, Kaiser's Eigenvalue criterion (>1) and Varimax rotation.

In addition to Classical Test Theory, the method of linear structural modeling was used repeatedly in the development of the ARSS. Hereby, the structural model and the measurement model were distinguished (Anderson & Gerbing, 1988). Linear Structural Models were evaluated by statistics of model fit. As recommended by Beauducel and Wittmann (2005), the following fit indices were used to evaluate the model adjustment: χ^2 and the corresponding p-value, *Comparative Fit Index* (CFI), *Root Mean Square Error of Approximation* (RMSEA), *Standardized Root Mean Residual* (SRMR), *Lower Limit of the 90%-Confidence Interval* (LO90), and *Upper Limit of the 90%-Confidence Interval* (HI90). As the χ^2 statistic is very sensitive to sample size, large samples will most likely show a significant result, indicating almost always that the empirically found model is significantly different from the hypothetical model. To prevent a possible misinterpretation, it is common to interpret fit indices instead of the χ^2 (Byrne, 2001). These fit indices and the critical values for evaluation of the model fit are given in Table 3.3.

Table 3.3 Fit indices to evaluate the model fit in structural equation modeling

Name	Short	Critical value	References
Comparative Fit Index	CFI	$\geq .90$	Beauducel and Wittmann (2005)
Standardized Root-Mean Square Residual	SRMR	$\leq .10$	Beauducel and Wittmann (2005)
Root Mean Square Error of Approximation	RMSEA	$\leq .08$	Hu and Bentler (1999)

The CFI is considered acceptable if it is greater than .90 (Beauducel & Wittmann, 2005). The RMSEA should be lower than .08 and the SRMR lower than .10 to indicate a good or very good model fit (Hu & Bentler, 1999).

The statistical analysis package AMOS provides modification indices to improve model fit (Byrne, 2001). These additional correlations were accepted in cases where theoretical arguments could be provided. They will be commented on in the text. For measurement models, correlated residuals (errors of measurement) were accepted if item content or formal item characteristics justified this correlation. This is, of course, a violation of the assumptions of Classical Test Theory – but it indicates characteristics of the scales. In the current manual, all analyses were run by AMOS in the SPSS package.

Note

1 At least three training sessions per week ($M = 10.7 \pm 4.4$ hours); regular participation in competitions (92%) [for more information, see Hitzschke et al., 2016].

4 The *Acute Recovery and Stress Scale*

Scope and application

The *Acute Recovery and Stress Scale* (ARSS) measures the current recovery-stress state of an athlete multidimensionally on emotional, mental, physical, and overall levels. It was designed to adequately present acute recovery-stress states of an athlete in a valid, sport-specific, and economical way. Coaches whose athletes complete the ARSS (in the morning after a supposed recovering night's sleep) will get information that is valuable for the daily training schedule and, if necessary, for adaptation of training. By regularly measuring the athlete's individual psychophysical stress state, overload symptoms can be identified at an early stage and in consequence, the performance control and training prescription can be optimized.

The ARSS can be used in sport-scientific practice, as well as in scientific research. Previous studies in Germany did not show any difference in perception and response bias for adults (Kellmann et al., 2016). With regard to the emotional items only, restrictions can be anticipated with adolescents (between 16 and 18 years).[1] These items must be interpreted cautiously or potentially cannot be interpreted at all. Whether they are evaluated depends on the individual case.

Sport-scientific practice

The ARSS offers differentiated information about the individual recovery-stress state of a person. The practicability in sport-psychological coaching has already been accounted for in the monitoring of several training periods in various types of sport. It can be used for the supervision of individuals, as well as for the supervision of teams and training groups. Cross-sectional and selective, as well as longitudinal, observations are suitable application settings of the questionnaire. Positive feedback was given from active athletes who used the questionnaire independently to regulate their own training, as well as from coaches who used the method for the monitoring of their entire training group. For the evaluation, a detailed profile can be created and reported back to the individual athlete.

Sport-scientific research

The ARSS can be used for different research questions in acute recovery and stress assessments in sport (e.g., to investigate the effects of different regeneration techniques). This applies to field and laboratory studies in sport psychology, training and exercise science, and sport medicine, and is especially helpful for high-frequency assessments.

Instruction

In addition to the appropriate questionnaire, this manual is needed for the implementation of the ARSS.[2] The following instructions are to be used for the ARSS:

> *Below there is a list of expressions that describe different states of recovery and stress. Please rate each item and mark the number that most closely applies to you **right now**.*

There is no time limit, and a strong habituation effect could be observed for the test duration. Depending on the familiarity with the questionnaire, the completion of the ARSS takes 4–5 minutes. To facilitate measurement comparisons over time, the ARSS should be filled in regularly and during daily assessments completed at the same time of day, if possible.

Evaluation

The ARSS consists of 32 adjectives that are answered on a seven-point Likert scale from '0' (*does not apply at all*) to '6' (*fully applies*). By calculating the mean value of the accumulated points from the adjectives, the scales *Physical Performance Capability*, *Mental Performance Capability*, *Emotional Balance*, *Overall Recovery*, *Muscular Stress*, *Lack of Activation*, *Negative Emotional State*, and *Overall Stress* are then formed (for exemplary items, see Figure 4.1).

The allocation of the adjectives to the scales is summarized in Table 4.1. In case of missing data, the mean should only be calculated when at least 50% of the items of each scale have been answered.

At the moment I feel / I am ...	does not apply at all						fully applies
1 recovered	0	1	2	3	4	5	6
2 muscle exhaustion	0	1	2	3	4	5	6
3 pleased	0	1	2	3	4	5	6

Figure 4.1 Sample items and answering mode of the *Acute Recovery and Stress Scale*

Table 4.1 Overview of item numbers of the ARSS scales

	Scale	Item number	Min.	Max.
Recovery Dimension	Physical Performance Capability	7, 15, 23, 31	0	6
	Mental Performance Capability	5, 13, 21, 29	0	6
	Emotional Balance	3, 11, 19, 27	0	6
	Overall Recovery	1, 9, 17, 25	0	6
Stress Dimension	Muscular Stress	2, 10, 22, 26	0	6
	Lack of Activation	4, 12, 18, 28	0	6
	Negative Emotional State	6, 14, 20, 30	0	6
	Overall Stress	8, 16, 24, 32	0	6

Note: ARSS = *Acute Recovery and Stress Scale*

Interpretation

The higher the value is on one scale, the higher is the current recovery or stress state in that area. Subsequently, there is some simplified information for interpreting the results. It should be considered that the values of the items differ strongly between individuals. A great dispersion is hence possible. All values should be regarded for each person with reference to their intra-individual dispersion, i.e., their personal range which has been determined through multiple measurements (Hecksteden et al., 2017; Meyer et al., 2016). This is especially relevant for long-term monitoring of an athlete. Moreover, the context or time of measurement of the ARSS must be considered. Particularly with regard to the overall and emotional scales, non-sport related factors can have a strong impact. Furthermore, the scale values can be influenced by the time of the day, as recovery values (as an example) are likely to be reduced in the evening of a day with a heavy training load. It is therefore recommended to record an individual baseline for each athlete (Hecksteden et al., 2017). These baselines should be established in normal everyday situations, ideally in pre-season or during a break from training and competitions, and preferably under identical conditions. For the interpretation of the item values, it is useful to collect additional information about training-related and non-athletic situations and events. That being said, another recommendation is to review developments in their chronological order and to check them for plausible changes of their values. Strikingly low values in the recovery scales and strikingly high values in the stress scales (over time) could be seen as an indicator for consultation.

Objectivity of assessment and interpretation is given, as the ARSS is a standardized tool with a method description of how it should be implemented and evaluated. Moreover, the objectivity of interpretation is obtained through the generation of a numeric value from the evaluation. Even though there are no norms for this tool, interpretation is possible as a high numeric value means an accordingly high value on the respective scales.

Recovery dimension

Physical Performance Capability

Athletes with high values on this scale feel strong, physically capable, energetic, and full of power. In training monitoring, this scale very sensitively describes recovery adaptations when using regeneration strategies.

Mental Performance Capability

High values on this scale suggest that athletes can concentrate well, are attentive and receptive, and feel alert. Context or time of measurement must be considered specifically with this scale. For instance, higher values can be observed in the morning, while lower values can be expected in the evening.

Emotional Balance

Athletes with a high value indicate being in a good mood, feeling pleased and stable, and having everything under control. The courses of this scale can significantly differ between individual athletes who experience similar stress and recovery stimuli.

Overall Recovery

Athletes with high values feel physically and mentally recovered and rested. In addition, they are muscularly and physically relaxed. This scale quickly shows reactions to recovery and stress stimuli. This more global recovery scale can reveal anomalies regarding influencing factors that are independent from sport and training.

Stress dimension

Muscular Stress

High values in this scale suggest that athletes feel their muscles to be exhausted, fatigued, sore, and stiff. This scale sensitively depicts preceding stress, but also stress reduction and recovery effects.

Lack of Activation

Athletes with high values on this scale feel unmotivated and sluggish, are unenthusiastic, and lack energy in general. The scale tends to show a reaction to long-term stress factors. Changes in the scale (both decreasing and increasing values) usually take longer to show than in the scales *Muscular Stress* and *Overall Stress*.

Negative Emotional State

High values point towards athletes feeling emotionally stressed by their current demand. They feel down, stressed, annoyed, and short-tempered. Depending on their personal situation, identical stressors can lead to a different experience of stress on the emotional level of each individual athlete.

Overall Stress

Athletes with high values in this area feel tired and overloaded, and perceive themselves as physically exhausted and worn-out. This scale sensitively displays changes in stress perception in relation to the stimuli. Like *Overall Recovery*, this scale assesses a more global aspect of stress.

Reference values and scale statistics

The ARSS was constructed in accordance with the Classical Test Theory (classical-latent-additive model; Moosbrugger, 1982). Therefore, an interpretation of the scale mean as an absolute value is not possible. Hence, the interpretation of the ARSS profile should refer to either a reference group of the athlete, to intra-individual changes over time, or to the mean and variability of single samples. Moreover, it is important to check whether the time of assessment corresponds to the respective comparison group. The psychometric properties of the presented studies will be summarized in the following sections. It must explicitly be emphasized that there are no norms for this questionnaire, and the creation of such is not intended.

The recovery-stress state varies during training camps, cycles of competitions, training weeks of the year, and different phases of life, as a result of specific stress and recovery activities. Therefore, the provided data in Table 4.2 have been collected in various situations (e.g., before training, after training, in-season, off-season) and should be interpreted as a reference value rather than as a norm.

Despite the circumstances just mentioned, the accumulated empirical results show overall central tendencies in the items, which are sensitive to change, but also seem to be typical under 'normal conditions'; thus, it was decided to calculate sample reference values. For the English sample, ES2 reference values were calculated that can serve as a rough orientation (Table 4.2).

The item-total correlation (r_{it} = .53–.78) of the English adjectives (items), the item mean (M = 1.51–4.35) and the item dispersion (SD = 1.29–1.80) were satisfactory for sample ES2. This supports previous results of the first English validation (ES1, see Appendix ARSS 1), as well as of the German ARSS (for sample GS3, see Appendix ARSS 2). Comparing the subsamples descriptively, it can be seen that the North American subsample showed the highest recovery and lowest stress means as well as a slightly higher item-total correlation.

Reliability

Homogeneity

Table 4.3 presents all construction samples, especially those with a target population as in ES1 and ES2, and shows a good scale homogeneity for the English ARSS (ES1 α = .76–.86; ES2 α = .77–.88). All language regions showed good scale homogeneity, but a slightly higher Cronbach's α was measured in the North American subsample.

The German sample GS5 showed slightly smaller yet still acceptable scale homogeneities for the adolescent male and female handball players. Cronbach's α ranged from .57 to .82 in the *Recovery* dimension and from .60 to .81 in the *Stress* dimension. However, low values for *Emotional Balance* (α = .57) and *Negative Emotional State* (α = .60) were apparent in GS5. This was also the case when the analysis was run separately for gender. Therefore, before future research supports otherwise, it is recommended to interpret these scales cautiously for adolescents or to not interpret them at all for this age group. A clear gender difference can only be observed in the scale *Lack of Activation*. This scale shows a lower scale homogeneity within the boys' group (α = .61 vs. α = .82).

Table 4.4 contains the changes in ARSS homogeneity over time for the subsample ES2_NA_II. While Cronbach's α showed a good scale homogeneity for the first measurement, an increase was observed throughout the assessments, with a peak at T5. As a rule, internal consistency increases with the familiarity of the individual with the instrument. Consequently, an introductory measurement is recommended for its applied use, as well as for research questions with repeated measurements, so that athletes can become accustomed to the ARSS. This finding does not only apply to the ARSS, but also to questionnaires in general ('Socrates Effect'; Jagodzinski, Kühnel, & Schmidt, 1987). This fundamental issue of changes in the internal consistency of questionnaires receives little attention and is rarely taken into account in research designs. In repeated measurement studies, an increase in Cronbach's α over time can be assumed.

Test-retest reliability

Since the ARSS is an instrument that focuses on the athlete's state and is sensitive to change, a high test-retest reliability of its stability over time should not be expected. Table 4.5 lists the correlation calculations during the five-day training camp in sample GS4.

Table 4.2 Descriptive data of the ARSS for sample ES2 (N = 1,039) and the subsamples ES2_ANZ (n = 379), ES2_UK (n = 316), and ES2_NA (n = 300)

	ES2			ES2_ANZ			ES2_UK			ES2_NA		
	M	SD	r_{it}	M	SD	r_{it}	M	SD	r_{it}	M	SD	r_{it}
Physical Performance Capability	3.79	1.12		3.78	1.02		3.58	1.14		4.06	1.22	
strong	4.02	1.29	.70	4.03	1.22	.61	3.85	1.33	.71	4.20	1.35	.79
physically capable	4.35	1.34	.62	4.34	1.22	.62	4.13	1.43	.59	4.61	1.38	.65
energetic	3.51	1.38	.67	3.44	1.26	.63	3.29	1.39	.66	3.88	1.46	.72
full of power	3.30	1.43	.73	3.34	1.33	.73	3.05	1.43	.72	3.55	1.55	.76
Mental Performance Capability	3.84	1.11		3.82	1.01		3.56	1.10		4.22	1.16	
attentive	3.91	1.38	.62	3.86	1.27	.58	3.65	1.42	.56	4.30	1.41	.70
receptive	3.77	1.30	.64	3.73	1.22	.60	3.54	1.31	.62	4.12	1.35	.68
mentally alert	3.93	1.37	.69	3.98	1.25	.66	3.58	1.41	.63	4.32	1.35	.76
concentrated	3.74	1.36	.71	3.71	1.28	.69	3.46	1.41	.64	4.13	1.34	.78
Emotional Balance	3.90	1.19		3.98	1.07		3.64	1.26		4.10	1.25	
pleased	4.01	1.41	.77	4.12	1.32	.69	3.80	1.48	.79	4.11	1.48	.81
stable	3.94	1.36	.72	3.98	1.27	.65	3.66	1.39	.73	4.21	1.40	.75
in a good mood	4.21	1.35	.73	4.23	1.26	.69	3.95	1.48	.74	4.47	1.32	.75
having everything under control	3.44	1.53	.66	3.59	1.41	.63	3.16	1.60	.65	3.61	1.58	.69
Overall Recovery	3.29	1.21		3.35	1.10		3.10	1.22		3.48	1.31	
recovered	3.86	1.52	.58	3.83	1.37	.58	3.71	1.59	.61	4.05	1.61	.56
rested	3.07	1.55	.64	3.11	1.45	.59	2.86	1.54	.67	3.30	1.65	.64
muscle relaxation	2.97	1.47	.68	3.08	1.40	.65	2.77	1.43	.69	3.10	1.59	.68
physically relaxed	3.28	1.47	.67	3.37	1.36	.60	3.05	1.45	.67	3.47	1.62	.73
Muscular Stress	2.62	1.42		2.80	1.34		2.62	1.37		2.39	1.54	
muscle exhaustion	2.58	1.67	.69	2.72	1.54	.67	2.58	1.66	.64	2.39	1.81	.75
muscle fatigue	2.66	1.64	.78	2.88	1.57	.78	2.66	1.61	.72	2.37	1.71	.83
muscle soreness	2.59	1.71	.78	2.79	1.59	.76	2.54	1.69	.76	2.36	1.81	.82
muscle stiffness	2.66	1.65	.69	2.82	1.60	.71	2.69	1.60	.69	2.42	1.72	.67
Lack of Activation	2.03	1.29		2.08	1.22		2.18	1.32		1.81	1.35	
unmotivated	1.58	1.63	.59	1.57	1.59	.54	1.77	1.69	.56	1.39	1.65	.66
sluggish	2.32	1.60	.62	2.43	1.61	.60	2.44	1.63	.61	2.08	1.59	.68
unenthusiastic	1.80	1.62	.66	1.86	1.59	.60	1.94	1.67	.69	1.58	1.62	.69
lacking energy	2.42	1.62	.63	2.46	1.55	.56	2.57	1.65	.63	2.18	1.67	.71
Negative Emotional State	1.89	1.27		1.86	1.17		2.13	1.36		1.67	1.29	
feeling down	1.51	1.60	.59	1.45	1.49	.56	1.80	1.73	.59	1.26	1.55	.61
stressed	2.57	1.80	.57	2.45	1.70	.53	2.85	1.87	.61	2.33	1.81	.59
annoyed	1.61	1.49	.62	1.64	1.40	.63	1.76	1.61	.58	1.46	1.51	.67
short-tempered	1.88	1.68	.53	1.90	1.56	.48	2.13	1.84	.54	1.63	1.65	.57
Overall Stress	2.56	1.39		2.61	1.28		2.64	1.39		2.37	1.52	
tired	3.30	1.71	.68	3.41	1.59	.65	3.34	1.69	.65	3.09	1.86	.74
worn-out	2.36	1.65	.77	2.45	1.62	.74	2.44	1.64	.75	2.17	1.70	.81
overloaded	2.28	1.63	.64	2.28	1.51	.53	2.47	1.67	.71	2.05	1.71	.69
physically exhausted	2.27	1.63	.75	2.27	1.59	.70	2.30	1.58	.74	2.14	1.73	.83

Note: ARSS = *Acute Recovery and Stress Scale*; ES = English sample; ANZ = Australia/New Zealand; UK = United Kingdom; NA = North America

Despite the time interval between the measurements on day 1 being the smallest, there was a training session in between the two measurements (see Figure 3.2). Hence, the correlations were (as expected) not particularly high. The highest correlations were found between the measurements in the mornings of days 2 and 3. With increasing time between the measurements (day 1 to day 5), the correlations became rather low. Due to the small sample of 24 athletes, these theory-approving results should be interpreted with caution.

Table 4.3 Estimation of reliability (Cronbach's α) for the ARSS for German (GS2, GS3, GS5) and for English (ES1, ES2) samples and subsamples

			GS2	GS3	GS5			ES1	ES2			
					total	♂	♀		total	ANZ	UK	NA
	Scale	N	429	574	239	120	119	267	1,039	379	316	300
Recovery Dimension	Physical Performance Capability		.94	.90	.82	.81	.83	.83	.84	.82	.84	.87
	Mental Performance Capability		.89	.84	.77	.81	.75	.78	.83	.81	.80	.87
	Emotional Balance		.86	.76	.57	.53	.61	.76	.87	.83	.87	.88
	Overall Recovery		.88	.85	.79	.81	.77	.81	.82	.80	.83	.83
Stress Dimension	Muscular Stress		.89	.87	.81	.78	.83	.86	.88	.87	.86	.90
	Lack of Activation		.89	.86	.74	.61	.82	.77	.81	.77	.81	.85
	Negative Emotional State		.84	.79	.60	.65	.56	.79	.77	.75	.78	.80
	Overall Stress		.89	.88	.78	.83	.73	.84	.86	.83	.86	.89

Note: ARSS = *Acute Recovery and Stress Scale*; GS = German sample; ES = English sample; ANZ = Australia/New Zealand; UK = United Kingdom; NA = North America

Table 4.4 Estimation of reliability (Cronbach's α) for the ARSS for the sample ES2_NA_II (n = 109)

	Scale	T1	T2	T3	T4	T5	T6	T7
Recovery Dimension	Physical Performance Capability	.84	.84	.88	.87	.91	.89	.88
	Mental Performance Capability	.89	.86	.88	.92	.91	.93	.90
	Emotional Balance	.88	.85	.88	.85	.90	.84	.85
	Overall Recovery	.81	.78	.77	.84	.88	.84	.83
Stress Dimension	Muscular Stress	.88	.81	.86	.86	.89	.87	.88
	Lack of Activation	.84	.85	.89	.85	.91	.84	.88
	Negative Emotional State	.78	.75	.84	.80	.84	.83	.81
	Overall Stress	.84	.86	.86	.88	.89	.88	.85

Note: ARSS = *Acute Recovery and Stress Scale*; T = Time of measurement; ES = English sample; NA = North America

Table 4.5 Spearman correlations (r_s) for test-retest reliability of the ARSS scales for the sample GS4

	Scale	Day 1 (n = 22)	Day 2–Day 3 (n = 24)	Day 1 & 5 (n = 23)
Recovery Dimension	Physical Performance Capability	.43 [c]	.67 [a]	.11 [d]
	Mental Performance Capability	.50 [c]	**.74** [a]	.54 [b]
	Emotional Balance	**.70** [a]	.61 [b]	.47 [c]
	Overall Recovery	.49 [c]	.54 [b]	.39 [d]
Stress Dimension	Muscular Stress	.68 [a]	.50 [c]	.47 [c]
	Lack of Activation	.20 [d]	**.81** [a]	.45 [c]
	Negative Emotional State	.14 [d]	.33 [d]	.40 [d]
	Overall Stress	.49 [c]	.69 [a]	.39 [d]

Note: ARSS = *Acute Recovery and Stress Scale*; GS = German sample; Day 1 = Beginning of the training camp and measurement in the evening; otherwise measurements in the morning

[a] = $p < .001$
[b] = $p < .01$
[c] = $p < .05$
[d] = non-significant; $r \geq .70$ are bolded

Table 4.6 Spearman correlations (r_s) for test-retest of measurement T1 with measurements T2–T7 for the ARSS scales of sample ES2_NA_II ($n = 109$)

	Scale	T2	T3	T4	T5	T6	T7
Recovery Dimension	Physical Performance Capability	.54 [a]	.63 [a]	.47 [a]	.64 [a]	.47 [a]	.46 [a]
	Mental Performance Capability	.49 [a]	.60 [a]	.56 [a]	.66 [a]	.52 [a]	.56 [a]
	Emotional Balance	.34 [a]	.60 [a]	.48 [a]	.64 [a]	.45 [a]	.40 [a]
	Overall Recovery	.20 [d]	.48 [a]	.29 [a]	.42 [a]	.21 [a]	.40 [a]
Stress Dimension	Muscular Stress	.06 [d]	.34 [b]	.25 [c]	.43 [a]	.24 [c]	.36 [a]
	Lack of Activation	.43 [a]	**.70** [a]	.59 [a]	**.74** [a]	.58 [a]	.52 [a]
	Negative Emotional State	.44 [a]	.64 [a]	.61 [a]	.57 [a]	.51 [a]	.59 [a]
	Overall Stress	.30 [b]	.53 [a]	.42 [a]	.61 [a]	.38 [a]	.44 [a]

Note: ARSS = *Acute Recovery and Stress Scale*; T = Time of measurement; ES = English sample; NA = North America

[a] = $p < .001$
[b] = $p < .01$
[c] = $p < .05$
[d] = non-significant; $r \geq .70$ are bolded

Another test-retest from T1 to T7 took place in a study on regeneration methods and the correlations for subsample ES2_NA_II revealed an expected pattern with a moderate range of the correlations (Table 4.6). T1, T3, and T5 took place before training and therefore are considered somewhat identical assessment conditions. In other words, under similar conditions (e.g., T1 and T3), the correlations were higher compared to dissimilar ones (e.g., T1 and T2).

Construct validity

Construct validity has been studied with respect to the intercorrelations of ARSS scales, the factorial structure, linear structure modeling, and the stability of the intercorrelations across different samples. Relationships to mood states, Delayed-Onset Muscle Soreness, and other criteria are covered in the section on convergent and discriminant validity.

Scale intercorrelations

The height of the scale intercorrelations proved to be similar across different samples. The fundamental correlation pattern was almost unchanged across all German and English samples and subsamples with respect to *Stress* and *Recovery* dimensions.

Based on the Spearman correlation coefficient, scale intercorrelations within the dimensions ranged from $r_s = .38$ to $r_s = .63$ for *Recovery* and from $r_s = .29$ to $r_s = .68$ for *Stress* for sample ES1. Correlations from $r_s = -.11$ to $r_s = -.64$ (Table 4.7) were measured between the scales of the *Recovery* and *Stress* dimensions.

Sample ES2 showed higher correlations within the *Recovery* and *Stress* dimensions, ranging from $r_s = .50$ to $r_s = .72$ for *Recovery* and from $r_s = .30$ to $r_s = .71$ for *Stress*. Correlations from $r_s = -.14$ to $r_s = -.64$ were found between the dimensions of *Recovery* and *Stress* (Table 4.7). However, as seen in Table 4.8, the North American subsample consistently showed the highest scale intercorrelations of the three subsamples (Australia/New Zealand, United Kingdom, North America).

The intercorrelation range of the English samples is similar to that of the German ARSS, which shows scale intercorrelations from $r_s = .46$ to $r_s = .71$ within the dimension of *Recovery* and $r_s = .19$ to .75 within the *Stress* dimension. Between the dimensions of *Recovery* and *Stress*, correlations from $r_s = -.21$ to $r_s = -.80$ were observed (for sample GS3, see Appendix ARSS 3). Slightly lower correlations between the dimensions of *Recovery* and *Stress* were measured in sample GS5 (see Appendix ARSS 3).

Table 4.7 Spearman correlations (r_s) within the ARSS scales for samples ES1 ($N = 267$) and ES2 ($N = 1,039$)

		Upper data matrix: ES2							
	Scale	PPC	MPC	EB	OR	MS	LA	NES	OS
Recovery Dimension	Physical Performance Capability		.72 [a]	.70 [a]	.58 [a]	−.23 [a]	−.60 [a]	−.43 [a]	−.50 [a]
	Mental Performance Capability	.57 [a]		.69 [a]	.50 [a]	−.15 [a]	−.56 [a]	−.43 [a]	−.43 [a]
	Emotional Balance	.63 [a]	.60 [a]		.50 [a]	−.14 [a]	−.56 [a]	−.64 [a]	−.47 [a]
	Overall Recovery	.57 [a]	.38 [a]	.46 [a]		−.55 [a]	−.40 [a]	−.35 [a]	−.58 [a]
Stress Dimension	Muscular Stress	−.37 [a]	−.11 [d]	−.23 [a]	−.63 [a]		.35 [a]	.30 [a]	.60 [a]
	Lack of Activation	−.51 [a]	−.42 [a]	−.49 [a]	−.43 [a]	.44 [b]		.67 [a]	.71 [a]
	Negative Emotional State	−.44 [a]	−.44 [a]	−.64 [a]	−.36 [a]	.29 [b]	.58 [a]		.62 [a]
	Overall Stress	−.47 [a]	−.29 [c]	−.41 [a]	−.64 [a]	.68 [b]	.64 [a]	.53 [a]	
						Lower data matrix: ES1			

Note: ARSS = *Acute Recovery and Stress Scale*; PPC = *Physical Performance Capability*; MPC = *Mental Performance Capability*; EB = *Emotional Balance*; OR = *Overall Recovery*; MS = *Muscular Stress*; LA = *Lack of Activation*; NES = *Negative Emotional State*; OS = *Overall Stress*; ES = English sample

[a] = $p < .001$
[b] = $p < .01$
[c] = $p < .05$
[d] = non-significant; lower data matrix modified from Nässi et al. (2017a); $r \geq .70$ are bolded

Table 4.8 Spearman correlations (r_s) within the ARSS scales for subsamples ES2_ANZ ($n = 380$), ES2_UK ($n = 316$), and ES2_NA ($n = 300$)

	Scale		PPC	MPC	EB	OR	MS	LA	NES	OS
Recovery Dimension	Physical Performance Capability	ANZ		.71 [a]	.64 [a]	.52 [a]	−.21 [a]	−.68 [a]	−.44 [a]	−.54 [a]
		UK		.67 [a]	.65 [a]	.58 [a]	−.13 [c]	−.46 [a]	−.30 [a]	−.35 [a]
		NA		.77 [a]	.80 [a]	.66 [a]	−.36 [a]	−.65 [a]	−.52 [a]	−.59 [a]
	Mental Performance Capability	ANZ			.69 [a]	.42 [a]	−.13 [b]	−.63 [a]	−.49 [a]	−.44 [a]
		UK			.66 [a]	.51 [a]	−.04 [d]	−.42 [a]	−.34 [a]	−.32 [a]
		NA			.71 [a]	.58 [a]	−.30 [a]	−.61 [a]	−.44 [a]	−.53 [a]
	Emotional Balance	ANZ				.42 [a]	−.14 [b]	−.60 [a]	−.72 [a]	−.50 [a]
		UK				.46 [a]	−.01 [d]	−.48 [a]	−.57 [a]	−.33 [a]
		NA				.60 [a]	−.27 [a]	−.59 [a]	−.62 [a]	−.56 [a]
	Overall Recovery	ANZ					−.60 [a]	−.43 [a]	−.39 [a]	−.59 [a]
		UK					−.44 [a]	−.33 [a]	−.21 [a]	−.48 [a]
		NA					−.59 [a]	−.44 [a]	−.42 [a]	−.61 [a]
Stress Dimension	Muscular Stress	ANZ						.29 [a]	.25 [a]	.56 [a]
		UK						.35 [a]	.22 [a]	.59 [a]
		NA						.47 [a]	.43 [a]	.67 [a]
	Lack of Activation	ANZ							.58 [a]	.67 [a]
		UK							.69 [a]	.71 [a]
		NA							.74 [a]	.76 [a]
	Negative Emotional State	ANZ								.58 [a]
		UK								.58 [a]
		NA								.73 [a]
	Overall Stress	ANZ								
		UK								
		NA								

Note: ARSS = *Acute Recovery and Stress Scale*; PPC = *Physical Performance Capability*; MPC = *Mental Performance Capability*; EB = *Emotional Balance*; OR = *Overall Recovery*; MS = *Muscular Stress*; LA = *Lack of Activation*; NES = *Negative Emotional State*; OS = *Overall Stress*; ES = English sample; ANZ = Australia/New Zealand; UK = United Kingdom; NA = North America

[a] = $p < .001$
[b] = $p < .01$
[c] = $p < .05$
[d] = non-significant; $r \geq .70$ are bolded

Factorial validity

The German ARSS

The first step to elaborate factorial validity of the German ARSS was to conduct an Exploratory Factor Analysis in sample GS1. The Minimum Average Partial test showed a four-factor solution for the recovery and stress scales. While the factor of the stress scales explained 58% of the total variance, the factor of the recovery scales showed a 61% clarification of the total variance.

In accordance with study GS2 (Hitzschke et al., 2016), the calculations of the CFA in study GS3 showed good fit indices and a very good scale homogeneity for the *Recovery* model (χ^2 = 290.28, df = 90, p = .001, CFI = .96, SRMR = .04, RMSEA = .06, LO90 = .05, HI90 = .07) with its four scales *Physical Performance Capability* (α = .90), *Mental Performance Capability* (α = .84), *Emotional Balance* (α = .76), and *Overall Recovery* (α = .85). This also held true for the *Stress* model (χ^2 = 352.76, df = 90, p = .001, CFI = .95, SRMR = .06, RMSEA = .07, LO90 = .06, HI90 = .08), which consists of the four scales *Muscular Stress* (α = .87), *Lack of Activation* (α = .86), *Negative Emotional State* (α = .79), and *Overall Stress* (α = .88). In the verification of gender variance, the model fit for both subsamples (women and men) was replicated. For the sample consisting of women only, the following characteristics were calculated: *Recovery* model, χ^2 = 217.91, df = 90, p = .002, CFI = .95, RMSEA = .07, LO90 = .06, HI90 = .08; *Stress* model, χ^2 = 331.24, df = 88, p = .001, CFI = .96, RMSEA = .07, LO90 = .06, HI90 = .08. For the men's sample, the following results were established: *Recovery* model, χ^2 = 165.10, df = 90, p = .03, CFI = .97, RMSEA = .06, LO90 = .04, HI90 = .07; *Stress* model, χ^2 = 206.70, df = 90, p = .002, CFI = .96, RMSEA = .07, LO90 = .06, HI90 = .08. The final version of the German ARSS formed the translation basis for the English ARSS.

The English ARSS

ARSS VERSION APPLIED FOR ES1

The version of the English ARSS is comprised of four items per scale (see 'Development of the English ARSS and SRSS' section in Chapter 3). Finalization was realized by examining the inter-item correlations, conducting a CFA, and observing the resulting changes of reliability after removing items. The four items, which showed significantly lower correlations with the other adjectives, were removed from the scales *Muscular Stress* (two items), *Overall Stress* (one item), and *Overall Recovery* (one item). Their removal improved the scale structure as determined by the CFA. All four removed items showed the lowest inter-item correlations and factor loadings. In addition, the final four items of each scale resulted in the best model fit, reaching the cut-off values for at least three indices.

The model fit for *Muscular Stress* was acceptable, but by enabling a covariance between the errors of measurement for the items 'muscle exhaustion' and 'muscle fatigue', further improvements were possible. In addition to acquiring the final structure of the three altered scales (*Muscular Stress*, *Overall Stress*, and *Overall Recovery*), CFA was also used to examine the composition of *Physical Performance Capability*, *Mental Performance Capability*, *Emotional Balance*, *Lack of Activation*, and *Negative Emotional State*, and to confirm the established German model structure. All scales showed good or excellent initial model fit for at least three of the four indices, except for the scale *Lack of Activation*. This scale showed appropriate fit for the SRMR index. For CFI, however, the fit seemed to be marginal and the fit for RMSEA was also poor. An excellent model fit for all fit statistics could be achieved through modification indices that suggested several improvement opportunities by allowing the errors of measurement between the items 'sluggish' and 'lacking energy' to correlate. Deleting just one of the four items as a method did not improve the measurement model, but resulted in a poor overall model fit for the RMSEA fit statistic (RMSEA = .48). The initial measurement models for all scales and modifications for the scales of *Muscular Stress* and *Lack of Activation* are also portrayed in Appendix ARSS 4.

FINAL ARSS BASED ON SAMPLE ES2

The process of data analysis utilizing the CFA for ES2 was conducted in four stages. First, a decision was made regarding the two reserve items for the scale *Emotional Balance*. This was followed by the analysis of the model fit for sample ES2 (initial and modified model). Finally, the modified model was calculated for each language region to determine the model fit (Table 4.9).

Table 4.9 Results of the Confirmatory Factor Analysis of the English ARSS scales for sample ES2 and subsamples ES2_ANZ (n = 379), ES2_UK (n = 316), and ES2_NA (n = 296)

		χ^2	df	p	CFI $\geq .90$	SRMR $\leq .10$	RMSEA $\leq .08$	LO90	HI90
First analysis									
ES2 (N = 1,034)	Recovery	660.652	98	.000	.936	.040	.075	.069	.080
Initial model									
		χ^2	df	p	CFI	SRMR	RMSEA	LO90	HI90
ES2 (N = 1,034)	Recovery	597.03	98	.000	.947	.038	.070	.065	.076
	Stress	847.66	98	.000	.918	.054	.086	.081	.091
ES2_ANZ (n = 379)	Recovery	296.05	98	.000	.932	.050	.073	.064	.083
	Stress	415.13	98	.000	.894	.068	.093	.083	.102
ES2_UK (n = 316)	Recovery	292.39	98	.000	.931	.049	.079	.069	.090
	Stress	354.25	98	.000	.907	.057	.091	.081	.101
ES2_NA (n = 296)	Recovery	318.12	98	.000	.933	.046	.087	.077	.098
	Stress	388.78	98	.000	.910	.061	.100	.090	.111
Model specification									
		χ^2	df	p	CFI	SRMR	RMSEA	LO90	HI90
ES2 (N = 1,034)	Recovery	510.55	96	.000	.956	.036	.065	.059	.070
	Stress	644.66	95	.000	.940	.050	.075	.069	.080
ES2_ANZ (n = 379)	Recovery	257.12	96	.000	.945	.048	.067	.057	.077
	Stress	309.00	95	.000	.929	.062	.077	.068	.087
ES2_UK (n = 316)	Recovery	247.43	96	.000	.946	.046	.071	.060	.082
	Stress	275.34	95	.000	.935	.052	.078	.067	.088
ES2_NA (n = 296)	Recovery	308.53	96	.000	.936	.046	.087	.076	.098
	Stress	366.94	95	.000	.916	.059	.099	.088	.109

Note: ARSS = *Acute Recovery and Stress Scale*; ES = English sample; ANZ = Australia/New Zealand; UK = United Kingdom; NA = North America; Gray fields indicate meeting the aimed threshold; CFI = Comparative Fit Index; SRMR = Standardized Root-Mean Square Residual; RMSEA = Root Mean Square Error of Approximation; LO90 = 90%-Confidence Interval; HI90 = Upper Limit of the 90%-Confidence Interval

Two additional items ('pleased' and 'stable') were added to the scale *Emotional Balance* after the analysis of sample ES1. Consequently, this scale consisted of six items. Distinct improvements for the model fits could be determined in the first analysis by exchanging the items 'satisfied' and 'balanced' with the items 'pleased' and 'stable', respectively (Table 4.9). **All analyses presented in the manual for sample ES2 were conducted with the exchanged items which consequently represent the final English ARSS version.**

While the initial measurement model for the dimension *Recovery* (Figure 4.2) had already met the threshold for sample ES2, this was not the case with the model for *Stress* (Figure 4.3); especially when considering the CFA for the subsamples (Table 4.9). An initial model fit for the dimension *Recovery* could only be observed for the Australian/New Zealand and United Kingdom subsamples.

As a result of the less-than-ideal model fit, two modifications were approved for the *Recovery* dimension for model specification within scales. With two modifications, a good fit was obtained (Figure 4.4). The first modification was a correlation between the measurement errors of two items from the scale *Physical Performance Capability* ('strong' and 'physically capable'). The second modification was a correlation between the measurement errors of two items from the scale *Mental Performance Capability* ('attentive' and 'receptive').

In the *Stress* dimension for model specification within scales, three modifications were accepted to improve the model fit (Figure 4.5). Two modifications were correlations between the measurement errors of items from *Muscular Stress* ('muscle exhaustion' with 'muscle fatigue' and 'muscle soreness' with 'muscle stiffness'). The last modification was a correlation between the measurement errors of two items from the scale *Lack of Activation* ('unmotivated' with 'unenthusiastic').

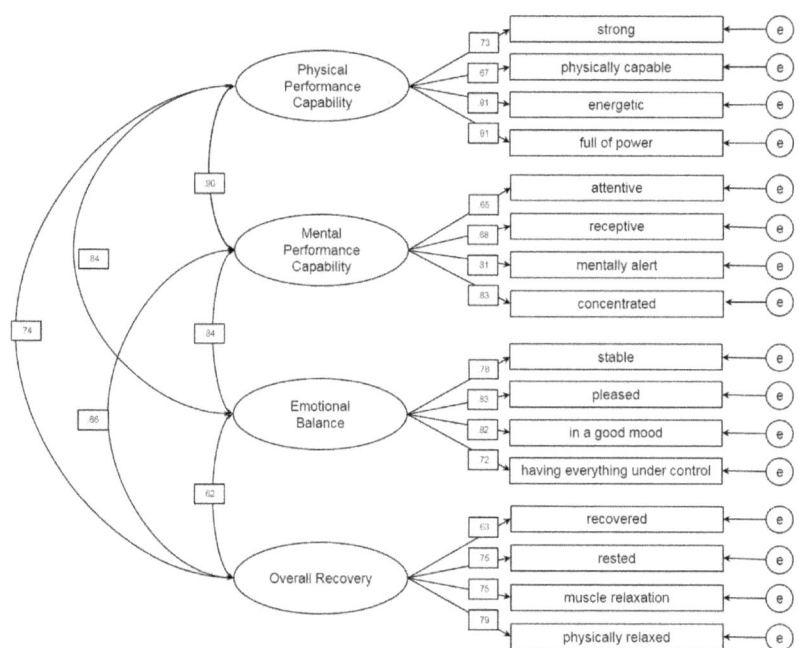

Figure 4.2 Initial measurement model for the dimension *Recovery* ($\chi^2 = 597.03$, $df = 98$, $p < .001$, CFI = .95, SRMR = .04, RMSEA = .07, LO90 = .07, HI90 = .08) for sample ES2 ($N = 1,034$)

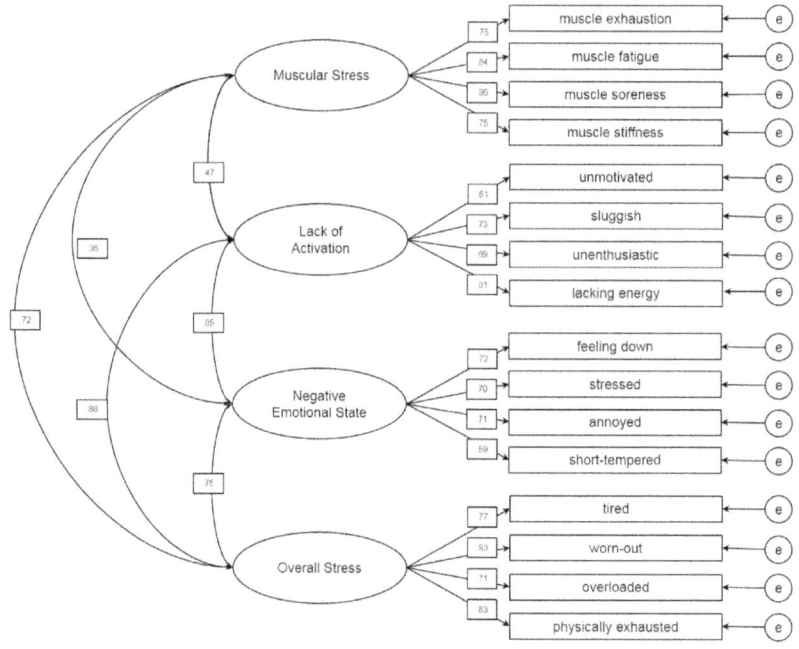

Figure 4.3 Initial measurement model for the dimension *Stress* ($\chi^2 = 847.66$, $df = 98$, $p < .001$, CFI = .92, SRMR = .05, RMSEA = .09, LO90 = .08, HI90 = .09) for sample ES2 ($N = 1,034$)

In further analyses, the same model specification of ES2 was applied to all language regions, which lead to an improvement of the overall fit for the recovery and stress models for the Australian/New Zealand and United Kingdom subsamples (Table 4.9). For the North American subsample, however, the RMSEA missed the recommended threshold.

Appendices ARSS 5–7 contain figures of the initial and modified models for the *Stress* and *Recovery* dimensions for the language regions. Comparing the modified models, it becomes obvious that the

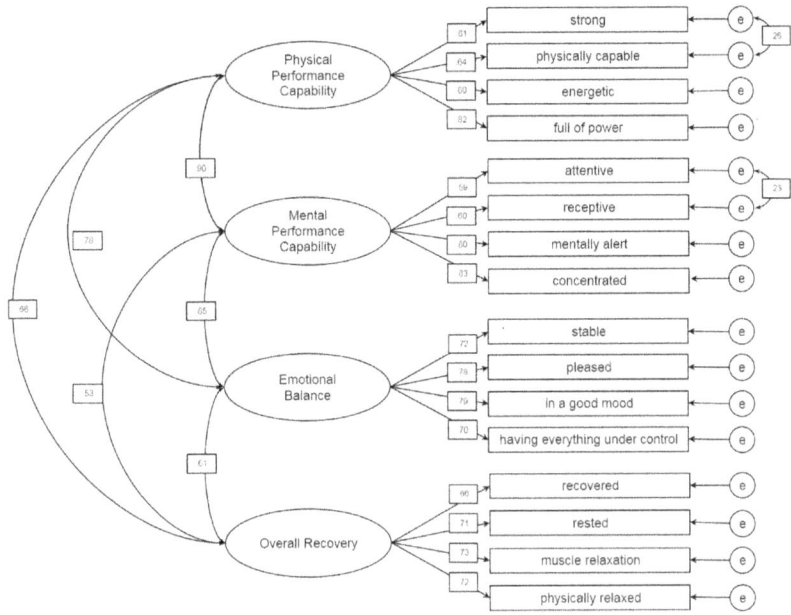

Figure 4.4 Modified model of the dimension *Recovery* (χ^2 = 510.55, df = 96, p < .001, CFI = .96, SRMR = .04, RMSEA = .07, LO90 = .06, HI90 = .07) for sample ES2 (N = 1,034)

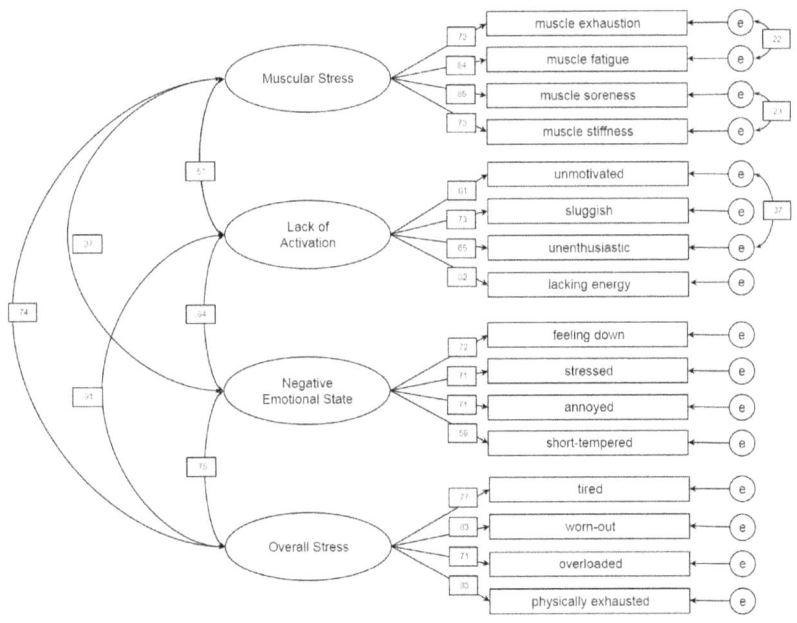

Figure 4.5 Modified model of the dimension *Stress* (χ^2 = 644.66, df = 95, p < .001, CFI = .94, SRMR = .05, RMSEA = .08, LO90 = .07, HI90 = .08) for sample ES2 (N = 1,034)

modification for *Muscular Stress* ('muscle exhaustion' with 'muscle fatigue') differ clearly between the subsamples (ANZ = .36; UK = .27; NA = −.17). This indicates that the understanding of these adjectives may differ between the language regions.

Overall, the CFA confirmed good model fits for the dimensions *Recovery* and *Stress* in the pooled sample ES2 and the Australian/New Zealand and United Kingdom subsamples. This result confirms the structure of the ARSS, even though the North American subsample is slightly over the recommended threshold for the RMSEA index (Brown & Cudeck, 1993).

There may be some explanations for the less-than-ideal model fit of the North American subsample. As pointed out earlier in the back-to-back translation process, we have experienced differences in the translation and interpretation of the adjectives due to the different English backgrounds. The final call on the items, however, was made by colleagues from Australia, who identified and modified items for the proper understanding in the Australian context. Based on language development, the Australian English tends to be closer to the British understanding – even if there is some debate in the literature (e.g., Trudgill & Hannah, 2017) – than to the North American. This may explain why for the Australian/New Zealand and United Kingdom subsamples the model fits well. As opposed to this, the North American subsample showed the highest recovery means and total-item correlations, as well as lowest stress means (Table 4.2), highest Cronbach's α (Table 4.3), and the highest scale intercorrelations (Table 4.8).

Finally, we suggest conducting further CFAs for the North American region with different samples to understand the current less-than-ideal model fit. While we strategically planned the across-language data collection to calculate the model fit, we were not aware of any other questionnaires currently used in sport psychology and sport science that differentiate between English language regions. Therefore, we suggest that language confirmation across different language regions becomes a standard procedure for psychometric instruments – at least in those cases where the items are based on adjectives. Where behavior is assessed, different variations of English may be of subordinate importance.

Convergent and discriminant validity

The recovery-stress state was validated against a broad range of criteria, which covers psychological measures such as mood state, sensitivity to change and performance, as well as physiological indicators.

Correlations with actual mood state

The expected relationships between the actual state and the English ARSS have been empirically verified, which supports the validity of the ARSS. The relationship to the actual physical and psychological mood state has been covered by the correlations with the RESTQ-Sport-76, the DOMS, and the POMS.

RESTQ-Sport

Concurrent validity of the ARSS was assessed by examining the scores in relation to the RESTQ-Sport-76. All three German construction studies (GS1–GS3) and one validation study (GS4) showed correlations with the scales of the RESTQ-Sport-76. This confirmed the hypothesis that positive correlations among the related dimensions and negative correlations between the opposite dimensions for both *Recovery* and *Stress* should occur (Kellmann et al., 2016). Appendix ARSS 8 presents the Spearman correlation coefficients between RESTQ-Sport-76 and ARSS scales for German elite athletes (GS3). In comparison to the other scales, the German ARSS scale *Emotional Balance* correlated more strongly with the RESTQ-Sport-76 scales *General Well-being* ($r_s = .65$) and *Physical Recovery* ($r_s = .64$), and negatively with *General Stress* ($r_s = -.61$). *Negative Emotional State* (ARSS) showed the highest correlation with *General Stress* ($r_s = .63$) and *Emotional Stress* ($r_s = .64$); *Physical Performance Capability* (ARSS) correlated more strongly with *Physical Recovery* ($r_s = .68$) and *Being in Shape* ($r_s = .68$). The *Overall Recovery* and *Overall Stress* scales of the German ARSS showed the highest negative and positive correlations with *Being in Shape* ($r_s = .64 / -.60$), respectively.

Similar patterns occurred for the English samples ES1 and ES2 (Table 4.10). Positive correlations among the related scales and negative correlations between the opposite scales for both stress and recovery emerged.

For ES1/ES2, the English ARSS scale *Physical Performance Capability* and the RESTQ-Sport-76 scale *Being in Shape* showed the strongest correlation ($r_s = .71 / .66$). *Muscular Stress* for the ARSS showed the highest correlation with the *Injury* RESTQ-Sport-76 scale ($r_s = .52 / .56$). *Negative Emotional State* (ARSS) and *Emotional Stress* (RESTQ-Sport-76) demonstrated another noticeable correlation ($r_s = .64 / .73$). In addition, in ES2, *Emotional Balance* correlated with *General Well-being* ($r_s = .70$).

The described pattern occurred for all three language regions: the Australian/New Zealand, United Kingdom, and North American subsamples (Table 4.11). However, the latter almost consistently showed the highest correlations.

Table 4.10 Spearman correlations (r_s) of the English ARSS scales with the RESTQ-Sport-76 scales for samples ES1 ($N = 267$) and ES2 ($n = 572$)

ES1; ES2	Overall Stress									Overall Recovery			Sport-specific Stress			Sport-specific Recovery			
	1	2	3	4	5	6	7	8	9	10	11	12	13	14	15	16	17	18	19
PPC	-.35 [a]	-.30 [a]	-.27 [a]	-.19 [b]	-.29 [a]	-.32 [a]	-.41 [a]	.40 [a]	.33 [a]	.61 [a]	.45 [a]	.33 [a]	-.20 [b]	-.31 [a]	-.29 [a]	**.71** [a]	.43 [a]	.59 [a]	.40 [a]
	-.42 [a]	-.40 [a]	-.32 [a]	-.33 [a]	-.33 [a]	-.48 [a]	-.47 [a]	.49 [a]	.31 [a]	.61 [a]	.51 [a]	.34 [a]	-.27 [a]	-.35 [a]	-.30 [a]	.66 [a]	.42 [a]	.57 [a]	.47 [a]
MPC	-.32 [a]	-.27 [a]	-.35 [a]	-.19 [d]	-.16 [c]	-.24 [a]	-.28 [a]	.31 [a]	.25 [a]	.39 [a]	.50 [a]	.27 [a]	-.11 [d]	-.27 [a]	-.13 [c]	.35 [a]	.49 [a]	.30 [a]	.39 [a]
	-.44 [a]	-.40 [a]	-.36 [a]	-.33 [a]	-.35 [a]	-.51 [a]	-.43 [a]	.48 [a]	.28 [a]	.55 [a]	.49 [a]	.35 [a]	-.28 [a]	-.37 [a]	-.20 [a]	.51 [a]	.39 [a]	.49 [a]	.37 [a]
EB	-.52 [a]	-.46 [a]	-.46 [a]	-.40 [a]	-.33 [a]	-.41 [a]	-.45 [a]	.47 [a]	.34 [a]	.58 [a]	.56 [a]	.39 [a]	-.32 [a]	-.43 [a]	-.27 [a]	.60 [a]	.42 [a]	.51 [a]	.35 [a]
	-.60 [a]	-.56 [a]	-.45 [a]	-.44 [a]	-.36 [a]	-.51 [a]	-.49 [a]	.53 [a]	.44 [a]	.66 [a]	**.70** [a]	.44 [a]	-.31 [a]	-.41 [a]	-.22 [a]	.56 [a]	.45 [a]	.54 [a]	.37 [a]
OR	-.24 [a]	-.21 [b]	-.25 [a]	-.23 [a]	-.29 [a]	-.20 [b]	-.38 [a]	.27 [a]	.24 [a]	.41 [a]	.31 [a]	.24 [a]	-.23 [a]	-.24 [a]	-.33 [a]	.42 [a]	.24 [a]	.25 [a]	.08 [d]
	-.29 [a]	-.30 [a]	-.21 [a]	-.35 [a]	-.44 [a]	-.35 [a]	-.48 [a]	.27 [a]	.22 [a]	.49 [a]	.32 [a]	.34 [a]	-.30 [a]	-.26 [a]	-.47 [a]	.43 [a]	.20 [a]	.29 [a]	.16 [a]
MS	.18 [b]	.15 [c]	.20 [b]	.19 [b]	.25 [a]	.19 [b]	.32 [a]	-.20 [b]	-.11 [d]	-.23 [a]	-.09 [d]	-.09 [d]	.23 [a]	.23 [a]	.52 [a]	-.26 [a]	-.09 [d]	-.15 [c]	.04 [d]
	.17 [a]	.20 [a]	.17 [a]	.23 [a]	.34 [a]	.26 [a]	.38 [a]	-.13 [b]	-.04 [d]	-.24 [a]	-.10 [c]	-.17 [a]	.26 [a]	.24 [a]	.56 [a]	-.22 [a]	-.03 [d]	-.09 [c]	.01 [d]
LA	.44 [a]	.43 [a]	.39 [a]	.31 [a]	.38 [a]	.42 [a]	.39 [a]	-.32 [a]	-.22 [a]	-.45 [a]	-.38 [a]	-.30 [a]	.33 [a]	.45 [a]	.33 [a]	-.47 [a]	-.28 [a]	-.34 [a]	-.20 [b]
	.54 [a]	.53 [a]	.47 [a]	.44 [a]	.45 [a]	.61 [a]	.57 [a]	-.43 [a]	-.26 [a]	-.53 [a]	-.49 [a]	-.38 [a]	.35 [a]	.50 [a]	.37 [a]	-.55 [a]	-.33 [a]	-.45 [a]	-.34 [a]
NES	.62 [a]	.64 [a]	.58 [a]	.50 [a]	.42 [a]	.48 [a]	.48 [a]	-.33 [a]	-.31 [a]	-.51 [a]	-.55 [a]	-.41 [a]	.33 [a]	.46 [a]	.26 [a]	-.43 [a]	-.31 [a]	-.37 [a]	-.21 [b]
	.70 [a]	**.73** [a]	.65 [a]	.60 [a]	.47 [a]	.58 [a]	.60 [a]	-.39 [a]	-.37 [a]	-.56 [a]	-.61 [a]	-.48 [a]	.43 [a]	.54 [a]	.34 [a]	-.50 [a]	-.35 [a]	-.42 [a]	-.24 [a]
OS	.35 [a]	.36 [a]	.39 [a]	.33 [a]	.44 [a]	.39 [a]	.46 [a]	-.24 [a]	-.18 [b]	-.41 [a]	-.30 [a]	-.25 [a]	.35 [a]	.39 [a]	.39 [a]	-.38 [a]	-.18 [b]	-.28 [a]	-.10 [d]
	.47 [a]	.49 [a]	.40 [a]	.49 [a]	.58 [a]	.55 [a]	.64 [a]	-.31 [a]	-.23 [a]	-.51 [a]	-.38 [a]	-.39 [a]	.44 [a]	.50 [a]	.51 [a]	-.50 [a]	-.23 [a]	-.34 [a]	-.20 [a]

Note: [a] = $p < .001$
[b] = $p < .01$
[c] = $p < .05$
[d] = non-significant; $r \geq .70$ are bolded; ES = English sample

ARSS = Acute Recovery and Stress Scale; PPC = Physical Performance Capability; MPC = Mental Performance Capability; EB = Emotional Balance; OR = Overall Recovery; MS = Muscular Stress; LA = Lack of Activation; NES = Negative Emotional State; OS = Overall Stress; RESTQ-Sport-76 = Recovery-Stress Questionnaire for Athletes; RESTQ-Sport-76 scales: 1 = General Stress; 2 = Emotional Stress; 3 = Social Stress; 4 = Conflicts/Pressure; 5 = Fatigue; 6 = Lack of Energy; 7 = Physical Complaints; 8 = Success; 9 = Social Recovery; 10 = Physical Recovery; 11 = General Well-being; 12 = Sleep Quality; 13 = Disturbed Breaks; 14 = Emotional Exhaustion; 15 = Injury; 16 = Being in Shape; 17 = Personal Accomplishment; 18 = Self-Efficacy; 19 = Self-Regulation

Table 4.11 Spearman correlations (r_s) of the English ARSS scales with the RESTQ-Sport-76 scales for subsamples ES2_ANZ ($n = 239$), ES2_UK ($n = 126$), and ES2_NA ($n = 165$)

		RESTQ-Sport-76																		
		Overall Stress							Overall Recovery					Sport-specific Stress				Sport-specific Recovery		
		1	2	3	4	5	6	7	8	9	10	11	12	13	14	15	16	17	18	19
PPC	ANZ	−.36 a	−.32 a	−.28 a	−.31 a	−.32 a	−.50 a	−.43 a	.42 a	.31 a	.56 a	.48 a	.38 a	−.23 a	−.31 a	−.27 a	.56 a	.33 a	.44 a	.32 a
	UK	−.44 a	−.41 a	−.33 a	−.37 a	−.29 a	−.51 a	−.46 a	.53 a	.22 c	.65 a	.45 a	.29 a	−.27 b	−.36 a	−.24 b	.69 a	.37 a	.62 a	.53 a
	NA	−.51 a	−.48 a	−.39 a	−.37 a	−.38 a	−.43 a	−.54 a	.54 a	.40 a	**.70 a**	.66 a	.41 a	−.27 a	−.42 a	−.37 a	**.77 a**	.56 a	.69 a	.57 a
MPC	ANZ	−.47 a	−.37 a	−.36 a	−.34 a	−.35 a	−.55 a	−.43 a	.47 a	.28 a	.54 a	.50 a	.41 a	−.27 a	−.42 a	−.16 c	.46 a	.32 a	.43 a	.28 a
	UK	−.41 a	−.42 a	−.39 a	−.30 a	−.25 b	−.42 a	−.33 a	.52 a	.30 a	.58 a	.50 a	.32 a	−.18 a	−.33 a	−.09 d	.53 a	.42 a	.51 a	.44 a
	NA	−.46 a	−.43 a	−.36 a	−.32 a	−.39 a	−.46 a	−.50 a	.45 a	.28 a	.56 a	.52 a	.31 a	−.28 a	−.43 a	−.26 a	.56 a	.47 a	.56 a	.41 a
EB	ANZ	−.60 a	−.55 a	−.43 a	−.47 a	−.33 a	−.51 a	−.45 a	.51 a	.42 a	.65 a	.68 a	.48 a	−.30 a	−.42 a	−.22 a	.48 a	.38 a	.46 a	.25 a
	UK	−.65 a	−.63 a	−.54 a	−.43 a	−.31 a	−.58 a	−.45 a	.60 a	.36 a	.65 a	**.72 a**	.41 a	−.23 a	−.38 a	−.15 d	.53 a	.37 a	.55 a	.37 a
	NA	−.59 a	−.57 a	−.44 a	−.42 a	−.42 a	−.47 a	−.56 a	.50 a	.55 a	.69 a	**.75 a**	.44 a	−.32 a	−.45 a	−.27 a	.66 a	.56 a	.63 a	.46 a
OR	ANZ	−.33 a	−.35 a	−.25 a	−.42 a	−.47 a	−.38 a	−.44 a	.18 b	.24 a	.37 a	.32 a	.35 a	−.28 a	−.25 a	−.47 a	.31 a	.16 c	.20 b	.05 d
	UK	−.28 a	−.20 c	−.20 c	−.26 b	−.36 a	−.31 a	−.49 a	.31 a	.14 d	.52 a	.27 b	.28 b	−.19 c	−.19 c	−.49 a	.49 a	.06 d	.35 a	.14 d
	NA	−.26 a	−.31 a	−.23 b	−.32 a	−.41 a	−.35 a	−.53 a	.31 a	.26 a	.58 a	.39 a	.37 a	−.36 a	−.35 a	−.49 a	.52 a	.31 a	.36 a	.23 b
MS	ANZ	.20 b	.23 a	.22 a	.28 a	.42 a	.27 a	.37 a	−.05 d	−.06 d	−.16 c	−.06 d	−.18 b	.27 a	.23 a	.56 a	−.18 b	.01 d	.03 d	.08 d
	UK	.11 d	.06 d	.08 d	.03 d	.12 d	.11 d	.26 b	−.12 d	.01 d	−.24 b	−.05 d	.00 d	.11 d	.15 d	.49 a	−.16 d	.09 d	−.12 d	.07 d
	NA	.23 b	.28 a	.23 b	.32 a	.41 a	.36 a	.51 a	−.20 c	−.09 d	−.39 a	−.22 b	−.29 a	.35 a	.35 a	.62 a	−.35 a	−.16 c	−.26 b	−.15 c
LA	ANZ	.49 a	.42 a	.42 a	.35 a	.36 a	.55 a	.53 a	−.44 a	−.25 a	−.56 a	−.48 a	−.36 a	.27 a	.51 a	.33 a	−.52 a	−.35 a	−.38 a	−.27 a
	UK	.54 a	.54 a	.48 a	.41 a	.43 a	.61 a	.49 a	−.44 a	−.25 b	−.48 a	−.44 a	−.31 a	.27 b	.44 a	.23 c	−.51 a	−.20 c	−.46 a	−.30 a
	NA	.61 a	.65 a	.56 a	.60 a	.59 a	.66 a	.67 a	−.41 a	−.32 a	−.61 a	−.57 a	−.51 a	.47 a	.56 a	.47 a	−.66 a	−.41 a	−.54 a	−.44 a
NES	ANZ	**.72 a**	**.72 a**	.66 a	.59 a	.44 a	.56 a	.58 a	−.43 a	−.46 a	−.60 a	−.65 a	−.53 a	.42 a	.55 a	.30 a	−.47 a	−.40 a	−.40 a	−.21 b
	UK	.68 a	**.71 a**	.64 a	.53 a	.36 a	.54 a	.48 a	−.31 a	−.24 b	−.48 a	−.56 a	−.32 a	.27 b	.50 a	.23 b	−.44 a	−.25 b	−.32 a	−.17 d
	NA	.68 a	**.77 a**	.67 a	.65 a	.59 a	.62 a	.70 a	−.34 a	−.37 a	−.59 a	−.58 a	−.53 a	.49 a	.58 a	.45 a	−.59 a	−.37 a	−.48 a	−.30 a
OS	ANZ	.43 a	.42 a	.37 a	.46 a	.54 a	.52 a	.56 a	−.31 a	−.25 a	−.46 a	−.38 a	−.35 a	.38 a	.50 a	.49 a	−.45 a	−.22 a	−.26 a	−.12 d
	UK	.44 a	.46 a	.47 a	.38 a	.52 a	.51 a	.59 a	−.27 b	−.13 d	−.44 a	−.28 a	−.27 b	.36 a	.46 a	.43 a	−.49 a	−.10 d	−.36 a	−.18 c
	NA	.56 a	.58 a	.47 a	.59 a	.65 a	.62 a	**.74 a**	−.29 a	−.27 a	−.60 a	−.45 a	−.50 a	.54 a	.58 a	.59 a	−.58 a	−.29 a	−.44 a	−.27 a

Note: a = p < .001
b = p < .01
c = p < .05
d = non-significant; r ≥ .70 are bolded

ES = English sample; ANZ = Australia/New Zealand; UK = United Kingdom; NA = North America

ARSS = Acute Recovery and Stress Scale; PPC = Physical Performance Capability; MPC = Mental Performance Capability; EB = Emotional Balance; OR = Overall Recovery; MS = Muscular Stress; LA = Lack of Activation; NES = Negative Emotional State; OS = Overall Stress; RESTQ-Sport-76 = Recovery-Stress Questionnaire for Athletes; RESTQ-Sport-76 scales: 1 = General Stress; 2 = Emotional Stress; 3 = Social Stress; 4 = Conflicts/Pressure; 5 = Fatigue; 6 = Lack of Energy; 7 = Physical Complaints; 8 = Success; 9 = Social Recovery; 10 = Physical Recovery; 11 = General Well-being; 12 = Sleep Quality; 13 = Disturbed Breaks; 14 = Emotional Exhaustion; 15 = Injury; 16 = Being in Shape; 17 = Personal Accomplishment; 18 = Self-Efficacy; 19 = Self-Regulation

DOMS

The highest correlations with the German DOMS were found with *Muscular Stress* ($r_s = .59$) in sample GS3 (Table 4.12), which highlighted the construct validity of this scale (see Hitzschke et al., 2016).

Table 4.12 Spearman correlations (r_s) between the DOMS and the German ARSS for sample GS3 ($N = 574$), as well as the POMS and the English ARSS for sample ES2 ($n = 114$)

	Scale	DOMS	POMS						
			Tension	Depression	Anger	Vigor	Fatigue	Confusion	TMD
Recovery Dimension	Physical Performance Capability	−.32 [a]	−.54 [a]	−.49 [a]	−.43 [a]	.68 [a]	−.52 [a]	−.37 [a]	−.59 [a]
	Mental Performance Capability	−.19 [a]	−.55 [a]	−.52 [a]	−.40 [a]	.67 [a]	−.44 [a]	−.49 [a]	−.60 [a]
	Emotional Balance	−.19 [a]	**−.70** [a]	−.65 [a]	−.58 [a]	**.73** [a]	−.59 [a]	−.57 [a]	**−.76** [a]
	Overall Recovery	−.47 [a]	−.38 [a]	−.27 [a]	−.32 [a]	.38 [a]	−.43 [a]	−.23 [b]	−.41 [a]
Stress Dimension	Muscular Stress	.59 [a]	.07 [d]	−.02 [d]	.02 [d]	.04 [d]	.20 [c]	.06 [d]	.08 [d]
	Lack of Activation	.21 [a]	.64 [a]	.53 [a]	.44 [a]	−.52 [a]	.63 [a]	.53 [a]	.64 [a]
	Negative Emotional State	.09 [c]	**.73** [a]	.68 [a]	.69 [a]	−.54 [a]	.62 [a]	.61 [a]	**.77** [a]
	Overall Stress	.47 [a]	.55 [a]	.43 [a]	.40 [a]	−.44 [a]	.66 [a]	.44 [a]	.57 [a]

Note: ARSS = *Acute Recovery and Stress Scale*; POMS = Profile of Mood States; TMD = Total Mood Disturbance; DOMS = Delayed-Onset Muscle Soreness

[a] = $p < .001$
[b] = $p < .01$
[c] = $p < .05$
[d] = non-significant; $r_s \geq .70$ are bolded

POMS

The original English version of the POMS is a 65-item Likert-format questionnaire with intensity scales ranging from '1' (*not at all*) to '4' (*extremely*). The POMS provides a measure of general mood disturbances and six mood states (*Tension, Depression, Anger, Vigor, Fatigue, Confusion*). The same time frame ('right now') was used for the ARSS and POMS. Although the ARSS and the POMS apply different types of scales (frequency vs. intensity; Diener & Emmons, 1984), analysis revealed close and theoretically expected correlation patterns.

Tension, Depression, Anger, Fatigue, and *Confusion* correlated negatively with recovery-related scales, whereas for *Vigor*, a positive relationship occurred (Table 4.12). The stress-related ARSS scales showed a positive correlation with *Tension, Depression, Anger, Fatigue*, and *Confusion*, but a negative correlation was found with *Vigor* for ES2 (exception: *Muscular Stress* and *Vigor*, $r_s = .04$).

While the described pattern was consistent, the height of the correlation varied across the Australian/New Zealand and United Kingdom subsamples of ES2 (Table 4.13). Due to different group sizes, the thresholds for the level of significance were different. However, mostly higher correlations occurred for the Australian/New Zealand subsample.

Sensitivity to change

The ARSS's major aims are to record the current recovery-stress state and to sensitively capture the change in this state depending on the training, stress, and/or recovery conditions.[3]

Laboratory studies

In the laboratory study GS6, 23 trained cyclists and triathletes ($M = 28.8 \pm 7.6$ years)[4] filled in the German ARSS questionnaire every morning for eleven consecutive days (Hammes et al., 2016). Between days 2 and 7, the participants completed a high-volume endurance training with two training sessions per day. The intensive training was followed by a recovery phase from days 8 to 11. The training program aimed to exhaust the participants. The level of exhaustion was displayed using the 'Lamberts and Lambert submaximal cycle test' (Lamberts, Swart, Noakes, & Lambert, 2011). The analyses of the ARSS showed a clear

Table 4.13 Spearman correlations (r_s) between the POMS and the English ARSS for the subsample ES2_ANZ (top line, $n = 61$) and ES2_UK (bottom line, $n = 42$)

	Scale	POMS						
		Tension	Depression	Anger	Vigor	Fatigue	Confusion	TMD
Recovery Dimension	Physical Performance Capability	−.61 [a] −.27 [d]	−.50 [a] −.39 [b]	−.45 [a] −.29 [d]	.56 [a] **.74** [a]	−.60 [a] −.26 [d]	−.37 [b] −.27 [d]	−.64 [a] −.40 [b]
	Mental Performance Capability	−.61 [a] −.28 [d]	−.60 [a] −.30 [d]	−.40 [b] −.27 [d]	.66 [a] .59 [a]	−.48 [a] −.22 [d]	−.43 [a] −.38 [c]	−.64 [a] −.37 [c]
	Emotional Balance	**−.72** [a] −.50 [a]	−.67 [a] −.50 [a]	−.58 [a] −.45 [b]	.68 [a] .66 [a]	−.59 [a] −.40 [b]	−.50 [a] −.51 [a]	**−.76** [a] −.58 [a]
	Overall Recovery	−.34 [b] −.23 [d]	−.26 [c] −.09 [d]	−.19 [d] −.27 [d]	.36 [b] .23 [d]	−.49 [a] −.20 [d]	−.11 [d] −.18 [d]	−.39 [b] −.23 [d]
Stress Dimension	Muscular Stress	.11 [d] .09 [d]	−.06 [d] .10 [d]	−.09 [d] .15 [d]	−.05 [d] .10 [d]	.32 [c] .22 [d]	−.02 [d] .13 [d]	.09 [d] .15 [d]
	Lack of Activation	.61 [a] .57 [a]	.43 [b] .55 [a]	.36 [b] .50 [a]	−.43 [b] −.54 [a]	.65 [a] .53 [a]	.47 [a] .57 [a]	.60 [a] .64 [a]
	Negative Emotional State	.61 [a] .67 [a]	.55 [a] **.73** [a]	.57 [a] **.73** [a]	−.46 [a] −.45 [b]	.58 [a] .57 [a]	.47 [a] **.70** [a]	.65 [a] **.79** [a]
	Overall Stress	.54 [a] .32 [c]	.37 [b] .24 [d]	.32 [c] .27 [d]	−.43 [a] −.10 [d]	**.72** [a] .38 [c]	.34 [b] .34 [c]	.55 [a] .32 [c]

Note: ARSS = *Acute Recovery and Stress Scale*; POMS = Profile of Mood States; TMD = Total Mood Disturbance; ES = English sample; ANZ = Australia/New Zealand; UK = United Kingdom

[a] = $p < .001$
[b] = $p < .01$
[c] = $p < .05$
[d] = non-significant; $r_s \geq .70$ are bolded

increase in the scale *Muscular Stress*, with peak values after the six-day training period ($M = 4.1 \pm 1.4$) compared with the measurements under resting conditions on day 1 ($M = 1.0 \pm 1.1$) and day 11 ($M = 1.3 \pm 1.1$). The scale *Overall Stress* also showed an increase on day 8 ($M = 3.0 \pm 1.0$) when compared to day 1 ($M = 0.9 \pm 0.7$) and day 11 ($M = 1.1 \pm 1.0$).

Field studies

FIELD HOCKEY

The sensitivity to change in high-performance sport was supported in study GS4 in a five-day training camp of the female German U21 national field hockey team (Kölling et al., 2015). Every morning and evening, the 25 players completed the ARSS (for the structure of the training camp, see Figure 3.2).

A decrease in values in the course of the day could be observed for the recovery scales on the first three intensive training days, while the stress scales showed higher values in the evening (Figure 4.6). However, values on the *Emotional Balance* scale mostly stayed stable, except for the values on day 1, day 3, and the pre-post comparison. The same could be observed for the scale *Negative Emotional State*, although there was no significant difference in the pre-post values. The pre-post comparison also displayed a decrease in all *Recovery* scales at the end of the training camp and an increase for the scales *Muscular Stress* and *Overall Stress*.

As a hint for cross-validation, the stress caused by the training camp also became apparent through the pre-post comparisons of the RESTQ-Sport-76 scales *Physical Complaints* ($M = 1.6 \pm 0.8$ vs. $M = 2.1 \pm 0.8$), *Injury* ($M = 1.6 \pm 1.0$ vs. $M = 2.8 \pm 1.0$) and *Physical Recovery* ($M = 3.2 \pm 1.0$ vs. $M = 2.8 \pm 0.7$). In addition, an increase in muscle soreness when comparing day 1 ($M = 17.6 \pm 18.1$ mm) with day 3 ($M = 40.0 \pm 17.9$ mm), and day 1 with day 5 ($M = 39.0 \pm 21.0$ mm) was identified through the use of the DOMS (Kölling et al., 2015).

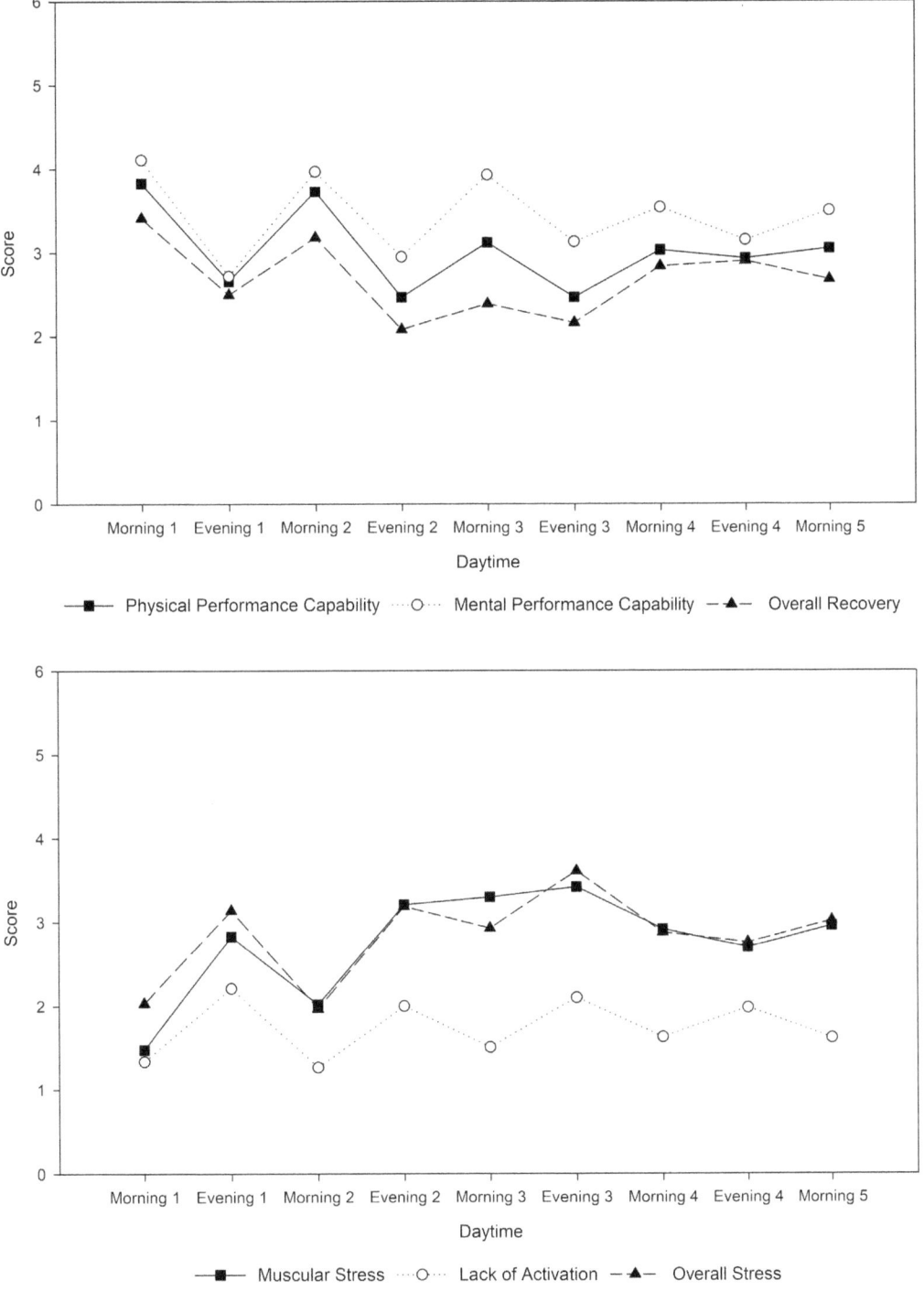

Figure 4.6 Three out of four recovery [top] and three out of four stress scales of the *Acute Recovery and Stress Scale* [bottom] throughout the training camp

Source: reprinted, with permission, from Kölling et al., 2015, p. 535

SWIMMING

The sensitivity to change and the applicability of the German ARSS for the individual athlete was shown by Collette (2016), who analyzed the data of nine female swimmers ($M = 19.3 \pm 3.1$ years) on a nationally competitive level. The ARSS was completed every morning during a period of 48 days, including a 16-day-long training camp. Athletes trained with a higher volume in this training camp, which led to an increased stress state. Concerning the ARSS scales, intra-individual changes and also strong inter-individual differences could be observed (Figure 4.7). The values on the scale *Negative Emotional State*, for example, were increased for two swimmers, while they were significantly decreased on another swimmer's scale. Opposite effects could further be identified between training phases for some athletes. The values did not decrease on all recovery scales and they did not increase on all stress scales. The training camp and the training parameters could still be classified as demanding, which could be derived from the ARSS.

Similar conclusions could be made after a longitudinal observation of the swimmers over a period of 152 consecutive days (Collette, 2016). With this observation, various structures of stress stimuli could be depicted from the different training phases. In addition, short-term and sensitive reactions to stress from competition could be detected. A pattern for the course of illnesses and injuries and non-sport related stress factors (e.g., stress at work) could be identified, too. The high linear interdependencies and cross-correlation coefficients proved the suitability of the ARSS as an instrument for long-term monitoring on an intra-individual level. The ARSS can therefore be used to observe the effects of training stimuli on the recovery-stress state.

Performance parameters

Hitzschke et al. (2017) aimed at investigating the effect of intensive microcycles in strength and high-intensity interval training on subjective measures of recovery and stress, and to descriptively compare these effects with variations among performance parameters. It was shown that the subjective perspective, measured via the German ARSS scales, reflected fatigue and recovery phases in a very sensitive and practical way, but could not exactly differentiate between athletes in fatigued or recovered states in relation to performance criterion measures. However, the descriptive data of ARSS scales and the counter movement jump as presented in Figure 4.8 indicate a correspondence of subjective and objective parameters.

Physiological response

Creatine kinase

Creatine kinase (CK) was chosen as a physiological parameter to assess information about muscle damage due to training. Several studies have tracked CK during training and competition as a marker of muscle damage or increased membrane permeability to the enzyme (Meeusen et al., 2013). Serum CK activity usually increases in response to strength training, especially due to eccentric exercise (Hortobagyi & Denahan, 1989), and normalizes when muscular adaptation occurs with training (Steinacker, Lormes, Lehmann, & Altenburg, 1998).

Two experimental studies, by Wiewelhove et al. (2015) and Raeder et al. (2016), were designed to induce functional overload in athletes by having them train at their individual maximal tolerable capacity. In total, 11 training sessions were completed (i.e., two sessions per day except for day 5; for a detailed overview, see Figure 6.1). During the experimental period, participants were instructed to maintain their normal dietary intake, which was recorded via food diaries, and habitual lifestyle while refraining from alcohol. No irregular dietary habits were observed, which was crucial for comparable conditions on testing days. Throughout the five baseline days and the three-day post assessment, participants were asked to refrain from intensive training or excessive physical activity. Moreover, participants did not apply systematic recovery strategies for the entire period.

The muscle damage due to training and its physical indicator CK was mirrored by the subjective rating of *Muscular Stress* and inversely related to *Physical Performance Capability* (Figure 4.9).

The present results suggest that a dose-response relationship exists between training load, CK, and the subjective assessment of stress and recovery. A high training load is indicated by elevated levels of stress and simultaneous lowered levels of recovery, which is supported by findings from Kellmann, Altenburg, Lormes, and Steinacker (2001) and those by Kellmann and Günther (2000).

Immunological responses

Puta et al. (2018) investigated changes of and associations between the German ARSS and capillary blood markers following resistance training in young track and field athletes ($M = 16.4$ years; range: 15–18 years) between morning and post-exercise sessions (112 observations from 13 participants), using Generalized

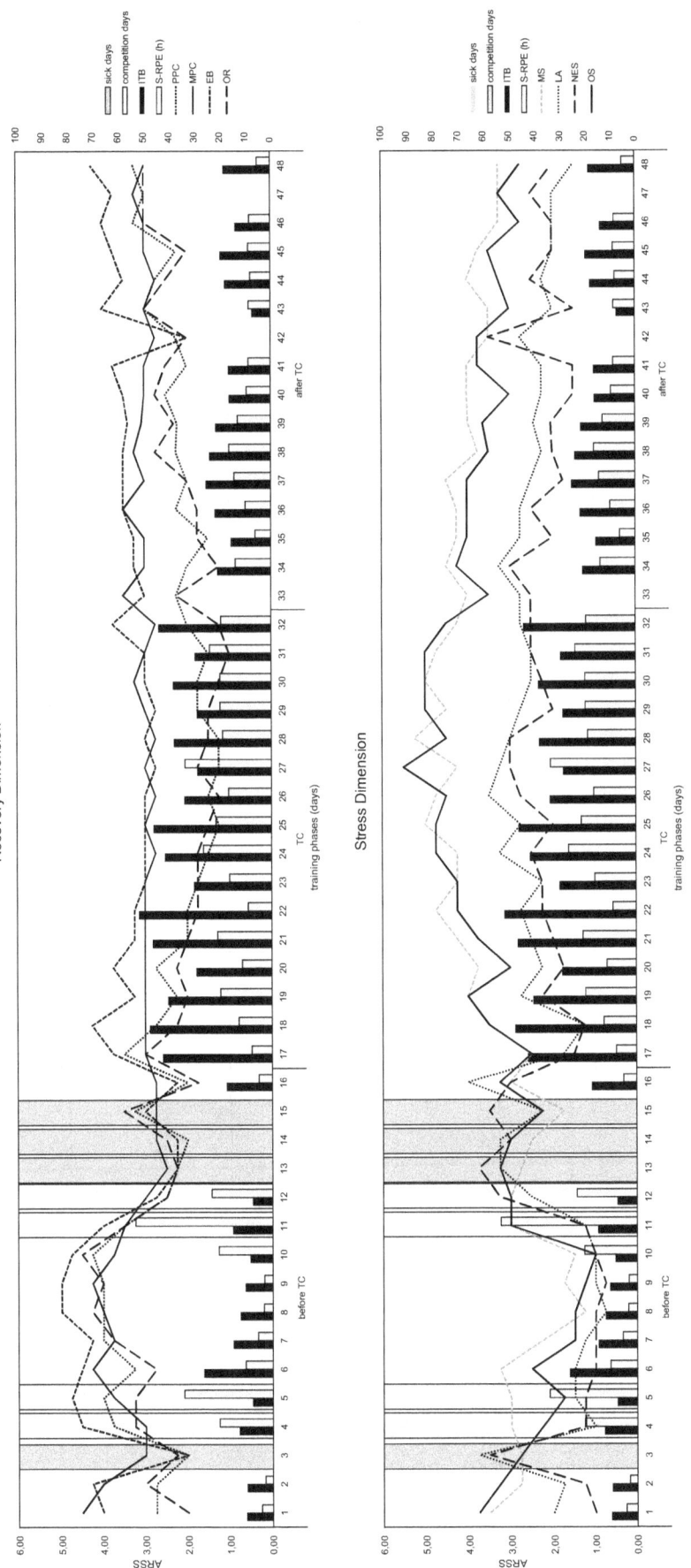

Figure 4.7 Changes of the *Recovery* [top] and *Stress* [bottom] dimensions/scales of the *Acute Recovery and Stress Scale* and individual training load (ITB) and Session-RPE (SRPE/h) over three training phases before, during, and after the training camp for athlete D1

Note: TC = Training camp; RPE = Rating of Perceived Exhaustion; PPC = *Physical Performance Capability*; MPC = *Mental Performance Capability*; EB = *Emotional Balance*; OR = *Overall Recovery*; MS = *Muscular Stress*; LA = *Lack of Activation*; NES = *Negative Emotional State*; OS = *Overall Stress*

Source: modified from Collette, 2016, p. 222

36 *The Acute Recovery and Stress Scale*

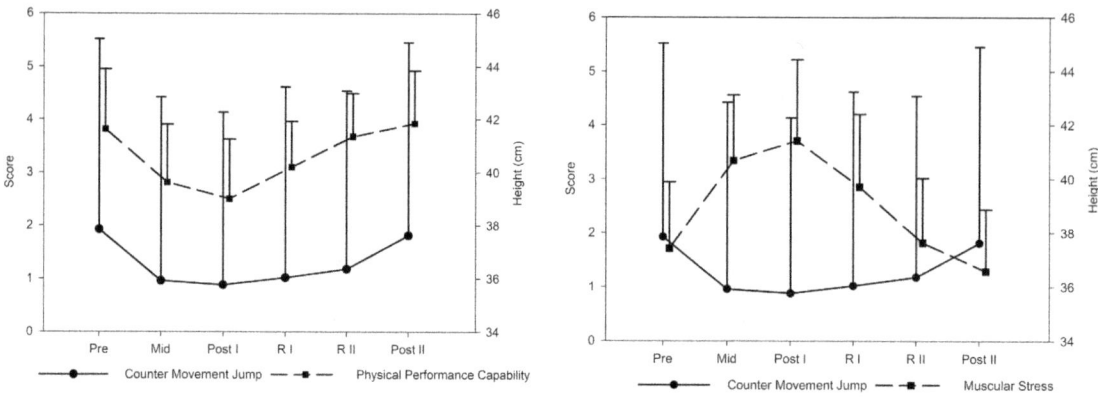

Figure 4.8 Changes of counter movement jump and the ARSS scales *Physical Performance Capability* [left] and *Muscular Stress* [right] during the study

Note: Pre = Pre-test; Mid = Mid-test; Post = Post-test; R = Recovery; ARSS = *Acute Recovery and Stress Scale*

Source: unpublished data from Wiewelhove et al., 2015 and Raeder et al., 2016

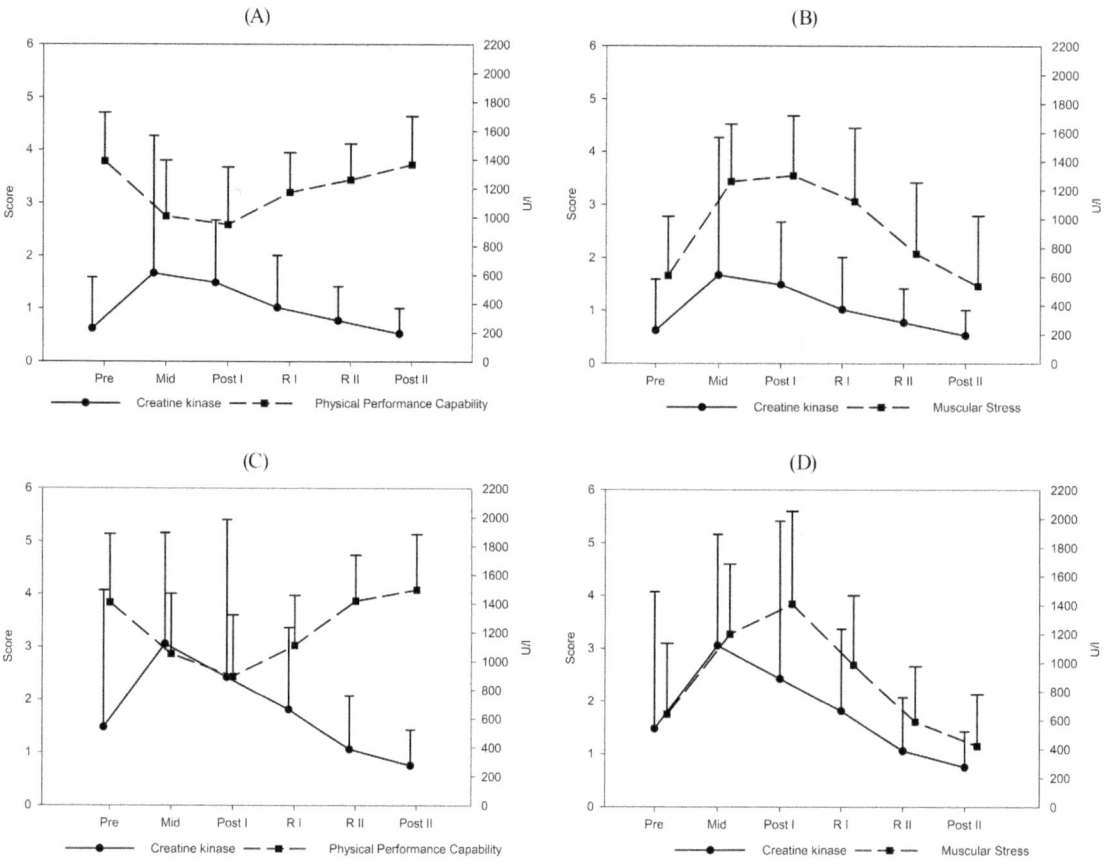

Figure 4.9 Changes of Creatine kinase (U/l) and the ARSS scales *Physical Performance Capability* [A] and *Muscular Stress* [B] for females and *Physical Performance Capability* [C] and *Muscular Stress* [D] for males

Note: Pre = Pre-test; Mid = Mid-test; Post = Post-test; R = Recovery; ARSS = *Acute Recovery and Stress Scale*

Source: unpublished data from Wiewelhove et al., 2015 and Raeder et al., 2016

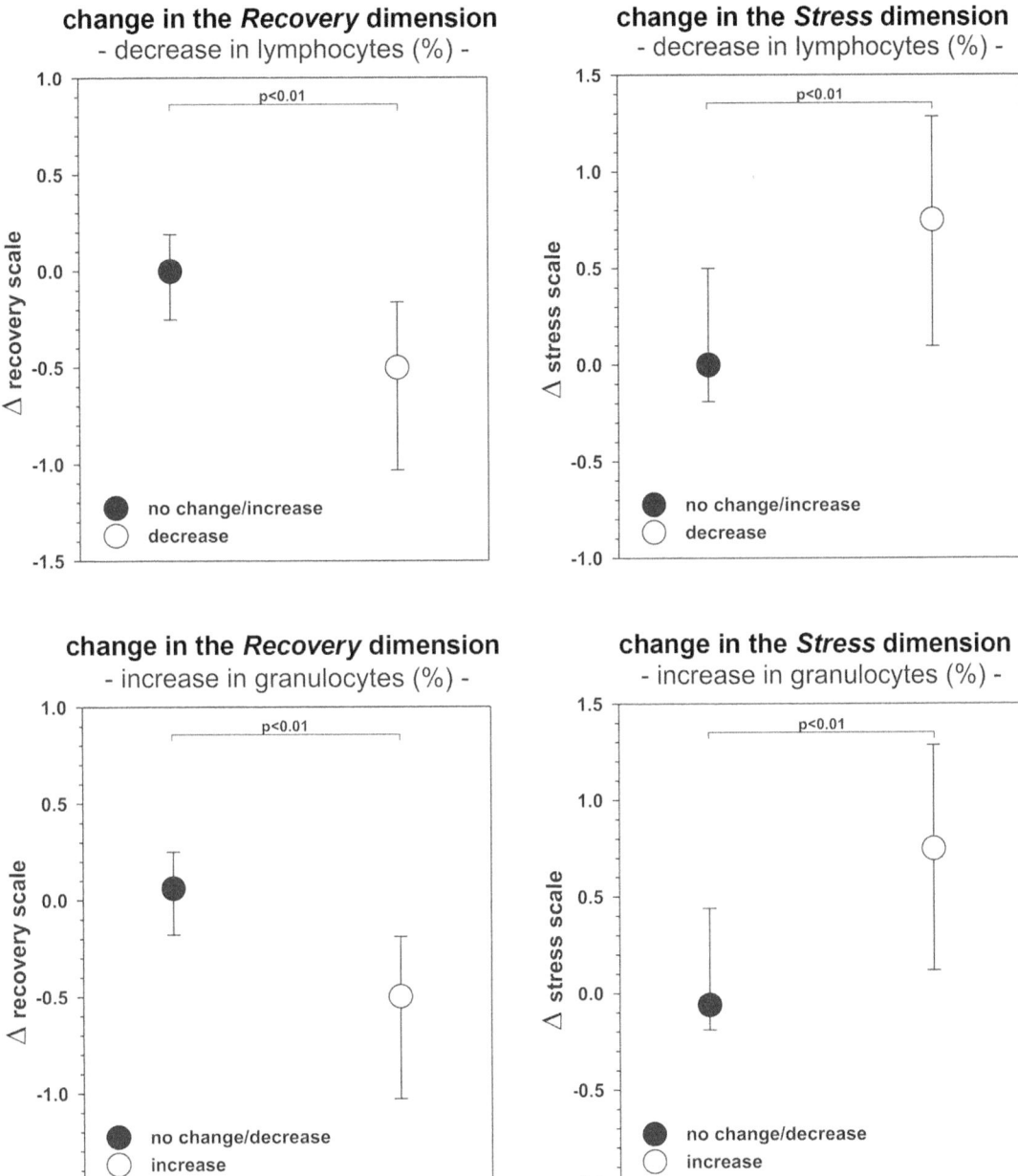

Figure 4.10 Median and first/third quartile (Q1/3) of the change-scores in the *Acute Recovery and Stress Scale* stratified by changes in percentage of lymphocytes and granulocytes. Bonferroni-Holm corrected *p*-values (*p*) of the Mann-Whitney-U-Tests are presented

Source: reprinted, with permission, from Puta et al., 2018, p. 7

Estimating Equations (GEE). In post-hoc analyses, daily change-scores of the ARSS scales were compared between participants showing specific changes in objective capillary blood samples. In the GEE models, recovery was significantly decreased, whereas stress was significantly increased between morning and post-exercise sessions.

Parallel to these measures, white blood cell count (WBC) and granulocytes (GRAN%) demonstrated a significant increase between morning and post-exercise sessions, while lymphocytes (LYM%) showed a significant decrease. Furthermore, using Multivariate Regression Analyses, it was identified that recovery was significantly associated with LYM%, while stress was significantly associated with WBC and LYM%.

Post-hoc analyses revealed significantly higher increases in the *Stress* dimension in participants who showed increases in GRAN%. Significantly higher decreases were detected in the *Recovery* dimension in participants with decreases in LYM% (Figure 4.10).

The experimental data demonstrate that resistance training is associated with exercise-induced immunological responses in young track and field athletes. More specifically, daily change-scores of the dimensions *Recovery* and *Stress* of the ARSS were associated with specific changes in objective immunological parameters (GRAN%, LYM%) between the morning and post-exercise sessions. The findings suggest that subjective manifestations of recovery and stress are related to objective measures of the exercise-induced immunological responses in young track and field athletes.

Summary of the ARSS

The ARSS assesses the current recovery-stress state of an athlete on emotional, mental, physical, and overall levels. It is a standardized self-assessment procedure and includes the scales *Physical Performance Capability*, *Mental Performance Capability*, *Emotional Balance*, and *Overall Recovery* in the dimension of *Recovery*; and *Muscular Stress*, *Lack of Activation*, *Negative Emotional State*, and *Overall Stress* in the dimension of *Stress*. The ARSS was constructed based on an expert survey and Exploratory and Confirmatory Factor Analyses. The latter confirmed good model fits for the dimensions *Recovery* and *Stress* in a large pooled sample (ES2, $N = 1,034$) and in the Australian/New Zealand and United Kingdom subsamples. The ARSS consists of 32 adjectives. The scales are generated by calculating the mean value of those adjectives, four adjectives for each item. The level of agreement is determined by a seven-point Likert scale ('0' = *does not apply at all* to '6' = *fully applies*). The ARSS is a reliable and valid instrument. Cronbach's α ranges for ES2 between $\alpha = .77$ and $\alpha = .88$. The convergent and construct validity is indicated through theory-conform relationships with the established instruments RESTQ-Sport-76, POMS, and DOMS under sport-specific stress and rest situations. The sensitivity to change could also be verified in the training monitoring of different sports which, however, still needs to be confirmed for the English version. Completion time for the ARSS ranges between 4 and 5 minutes.

Notes

1 Recent data of the German ARSS for a sample of children (10–13 years, $n = 312$) indicate that explanatory attributes for some items lead to a better understanding and in parts to a substantial increase of Cronbach's α. A similar effect also occurs for the age group 14–16 years (with additional explanation, $n = 441$; without explanation, $n = 303$), however, a substantial difference in Cronbach's α only occurs for the *Emotional Balance* scale. By the end of 2018, there are no substantial samples/data from children and adolescents available for the English version to support similar conclusions.
2 Please note: We strongly emphasize that the instruction, the order of the items, and the rating scale are used in their original form. Any modification or unauthorized translation into other languages constitutes a breach of the copyright and violation of basic research ethics (see also User information for the *Acute Recovery and Stress Scale* and the *Short Recovery and Stress Scale*).
3 So far, there are no validation studies which are utilizing the English ARSS, as this manual was published at the beginning of 2019. The final data analysis of sample ES2 was performed in June 2018.
4 Inclusion criteria: A minimum of 5,000 km of training volume per year; national (or higher) level of competition.

5 The *Short Recovery and Stress Scale*

Scope and application

The *Short Recovery and Stress Scale* (SRSS) measures the current recovery-stress state of an athlete multidimensionally with eight items on emotional, mental, physical, and overall levels. It was designed to adequately present acute recovery-stress states of an athlete in a valid, sport-specific and economical way. Coaches whose athletes complete the SRSS (in the morning after a supposed recovering night's sleep) will get information that is valuable for the daily training schedule and, if necessary, for adaptation of training. By regularly measuring the athlete's individual psychophysical stress state, overload symptoms can be identified at an early stage and in consequence, the performance control and training prescription can be optimized.

The SRSS was derived from the eight scales of the ARSS which were then grouped into the *Short Recovery Scale* and the *Short Stress Scale* and consist of four items each. The SRSS is an abridged version of the ARSS, which implies that the same changes during the development process that were made to the English ARSS were also applied to the English SRSS. No changes occurred in the actual items of the SRSS. However, the descriptive examples listed under each item were modified in the translation and data collection processes to match the structure of the ARSS. The scale labels of the ARSS are referred to as items of the SRSS. Each item of the SRSS lists the four ARSS adjectives as descriptors (see Figure 5.1).

Physical Performance Capability

e.g.
strong,
physically capable,
energetic,
full of power

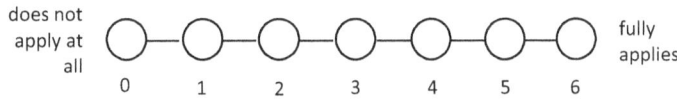

Figure 5.1 Sample item of the *Short Recovery Scale*

The SRSS can be used in sport-scientific practice as well as in scientific research. Previous studies in Germany did not show any difference in perception and response bias for adults (Kellmann et al., 2016). With regard to the emotional items only, restrictions can be anticipated with adolescents (between 16 and 18 years).[1] These items must be interpreted cautiously or potentially cannot be interpreted at all. Whether they are evaluated depends on the individual case.

Sport-scientific practice

In the sport-scientific practice, the SRSS offers differentiated information about the individual recovery-stress state of a person. This can be used for training regulation and to prevent overload and overtraining. The practicability in sport-psychological coaching has already been accounted for in the monitoring of several training periods in various types of sport. It can be used for the supervision of individuals as well as for the supervision of teams and training groups. The SRSS is suitable for cross-sectional, selective, and longitudinal observations. Positive feedback has been given from active athletes who used the tool independently to regulate their own training as well as from coaches and other officially involved persons who used the tool for the monitoring of their entire training group. Athlete information is easily and quickly obtained due to the compactness of the SRSS. When the scores are visualized on a board or screen, a quick assessment of the athlete's current individual recovery-stress state and the course over time can be provided. The SRSS helps to create a detailed athlete evaluation profile, which can also be reported back to the athlete.

Sport-scientific research

The SRSS can be used for different research questions in acute recovery and stress assessments in high-performance sport, e.g., to investigate the effects of different regeneration techniques. This applies to field and laboratory studies in sport psychology, training and exercise science, and sport medicine, and is especially helpful for high-frequency assessments.

Instruction

For the implementation of the SRSS, only the questionnaire is needed as test material.[2] When speaking of the test material in a broader sense, this manual is part of it. The following test instructions are to be used for the SRSS:

Short Recovery Scale: *Below you find a list of expressions that describe different aspects of your current state of recovery. Rate how you feel right now in relation to your best ever recovery state.*

Short Stress Scale: *Below you find a list of expressions that describe different aspects of your current state of stress. Rate how you feel right now in relation to your highest ever stress state.*

There is no time limit, and a habituation effect could be observed for the test duration. Depending on the familiarity with the SRSS, the completion of the questionnaire takes 40–60 seconds. To facilitate measurement comparisons over time, the SRSS should be filled in regularly and during daily assessments completed at the same time of day, if possible.

Evaluation

The SRSS consists of eight items (Table 5.1) that are answered on a seven-point Likert scale from '0' (*does not apply at all*) to '6' (*fully applies*). Forming the mean value of the *Short Recovery and Stress Scale* is **not** recommended since the response of the multidimensional items to training is different and, therefore, a mean value would overlay the response of the single items. Moreover, the CFA of the ARSS confirmed four separate dimensions within each model for *Recovery* and *Stress*. Lastly, the scoring, interpretation and evaluation should be performed on the basis of the single items only.

Table 5.1 Overview of the SRSS items

	Item	Min.	Max.
Short Recovery Scale	Physical Performance Capability (*strong, physically capable, energetic, full of power*)	0	6
	Mental Performance Capability (*attentive, receptive, mentally alert, concentrated*)	0	6
	Emotional Balance (*pleased, stable, in a good mood, having everything under control*)	0	6
	Overall Recovery (*recovered, rested, muscle relaxation, physically relaxed*)	0	6
Short Stress Scale	Muscular Stress (*muscle exhaustion, muscle fatigue, muscle soreness, muscle stiffness*)	0	6
	Lack of Activation (*unmotivated, sluggish, unenthusiastic, lacking energy*)	0	6
	Negative Emotional State (*feeling down, stressed, annoyed, short-tempered*)	0	6
	Overall Stress (*tired, worn-out, overloaded, physically exhausted*)	0	6

Note: SRSS = *Short Recovery and Stress Scale*

Interpretation

The higher the value is for an item, the higher is the current recovery or stress state regarding this item. Subsequently, there is some simplified information for interpreting the results. It should be considered that the values of the items can differ strongly between individuals. A great dispersion is hence possible. All values should be regarded for each person with reference to their intra-individual dispersion (i.e., their personal range which has been determined through multiple measurements; Hecksteden et al., 2017;

Meyer et al., 2016). This is especially important for a long-term monitoring of an athlete. Moreover, the context or time of measurement of the SRSS must be considered. Particularly with regard to the general and emotional items, non-sport related factors can have a strong impact. Furthermore, the items can be influenced by the time of the day as recovery values (as an example) are likely to be reduced in the evening of a day with a heavy training load. It is therefore recommended to record an individual baseline for each athlete. These baselines should be established in normal everyday situations, ideally in pre-season or during a break from training and competition and preferably under identical conditions. For the interpretation of the item values, it is useful and sensible to collect additional information about training-related and non-athletic situations and events. That being said, another recommendation is to review developments in their chronological order and to check them for plausible changes of their values.

Objectivity of assessment and interpretation are given, as the SRSS is a standardized tool with a method description of how it should be implemented and evaluated. Moreover, the objectivity of interpretation is obtained through the generation of a numeric value from the evaluation. Even though there are no norms for this tool, interpretation is possible as a high numeric value means an accordingly high value on the respective items.

Short Recovery Scale

Physical Performance Capability

Athletes with a high value feel strong, physically capable, energetic, and full of power. In training monitoring, this item very sensitively describes recovery adaptations when using regeneration strategies.

Mental Performance Capability

A high value on this item suggests that athletes can concentrate well, are attentive and receptive, and feel alert. Context and time of the measurement must be considered with this item especially. For instance, the value for this item tends to be higher in the morning and lower in the evening.

Emotional Balance

Athletes with a high value indicate being in a good mood, feeling pleased and stable, and having everything under control. The courses of this item can significantly differ between individual athletes who experience similar stress and recovery stimuli.

Overall Recovery

Athletes with high values feel physically and mentally recovered and rested. In addition, they are muscularly and physically relaxed. This item sensitively shows reactions to recovery and stress stimuli.

Short Stress Scale

Muscular Stress

A high value suggests that athletes feel their muscles to be exhausted, fatigued, sore, and stiff. This item sensitively depicts preceding stress, but also stress reduction and recovery effects.

Lack of Activation

Athletes with a high value feel unmotivated and sluggish, are unenthusiastic, and lack energy in general. The item tends to show a reaction to long-term stress factors. Changes in the item (both decreasing and increasing values) usually take longer to show than in the items *Muscular Stress* and *Overall Stress*.

Negative Emotional State

A high value points towards athletes feeling emotionally stressed by their current demand. They feel down, stressed, annoyed, and short-tempered. Depending on their personal situation, identical stressors can lead to a different experience of stress on the emotional level of each individual athlete.

Overall Stress

Athletes with a high value feel tired and overloaded, and perceive themselves as physically exhausted and worn-out. This item sensitively displays changes in stress perception in relation to the stimuli. Like *Overall Recovery*, this item assesses a more global aspect of stress.

Reference values and item statistics

As with the ARSS, the interpretation of the SRSS profile should refer to either a reference group of the athlete, to intra-individual changes over time, or to the mean and variability of single samples. Moreover, it is important to check whether the time of assessment corresponds to the respective comparison group. The psychometric properties from the presented studies will be summarized in the following sections. It must be explicitly emphasized that there are no norms for this instrument, and the creation of such is not intended.

The recovery-stress state varies during training camps, cycles of competitions, training weeks of the year, and different phases of life, as a result of specific stress and recovery activities. Therefore, the provided data in Table 5.2 have been collected in various situations (e.g., before training, after training, in-season, off-season) and as a result, should be interpreted as a reference value rather than as a norm.

Despite the circumstances previously mentioned, the accumulated empirical results show overall central tendencies in the items, which are sensitive to change, but also seem to be typical under 'normal conditions'; thus, it was decided to calculate sample reference values. For the English sample, ES2 reference values were calculated that can serve as a rough orientation (Table 5.2).

Table 5.2 Descriptive data of the SRSS for samples ES2 ($N = 907$) and subsamples ES2_ANZ ($n = 368$), ES2_UK ($n = 304$), and ES2_NA ($n = 186$)

	Item	ES2			ES2_ANZ			ES2_UK			ES2_NA		
		M	SD	r_{it}	M	SD	r_{it}	M	SD	r_{it}	M	SD	r_{it}
Short Recovery Scale	Physical Performance Capability	3.89	1.22	.69	3.88	1.17	.69	3.76	1.17	.63	4.16	1.39	.77
	Mental Performance Capability	3.96	1.27	.72	3.89	1.23	.72	3.81	1.29	.69	4.42	1.25	.77
	Emotional Balance	3.87	1.34	.67	3.92	1.28	.67	3.62	1.39	.60	4.20	1.37	.73
	Overall Recovery	3.65	1.26	.64	3.69	1.23	.62	3.45	1.22	.63	3.89	1.37	.66
Short Stress Scale	Muscular Stress	2.76	1.55	.34	2.84	1.52	.32	2.80	1.49	.31	2.55	1.72	.41
	Lack of Activation	2.24	1.51	.66	2.29	1.50	.60	2.34	1.46	.67	1.90	1.57	.76
	Negative Emotional State	2.10	1.63	.61	2.05	1.58	.61	2.33	1.65	.56	1.84	1.70	.67
	Overall Stress	2.53	1.52	.75	2.48	1.49	.73	2.65	1.41	.75	2.36	1.76	.80

Note: SRSS = *Short Recovery and Stress Scale*; ES = English sample; ANZ = Australia/New Zealand; UK = United Kingdom; NA = North America

The item-total correlation ($r_{it} = .34–.75$) of the SRSS (ES2), the item mean ($M = 2.10–3.96$), and the item dispersion ($SD = 1.22–1.63$) were satisfactory. This supports previous results of the first English validation (ES1, see Appendix SRSS 1) and of the German SRSS (see Appendix SRSS 2). Comparing the subsamples, it can be seen that the North American subsample showed the highest recovery and lowest stress scores, as well as a slightly higher item-total correlation.

Reliability

Homogeneity

The SRSS confirmed good homogeneity for the *Short Recovery Scale* and the *Short Stress Scale* regarding internal consistency for samples ES1 and ES2 (Table 5.3). Similar values occurred for the German sample GS3. All language regions showed good scale homogeneity, but a slightly higher Cronbach's α was measured in the North American subsample.

Nevertheless, it has to be noted that Cronbach's α is not an important criterion for the quality of the psychometric properties in this case, because scale homogeneity calculations for the SRSS are structure- and content-wise not relevant. On the item level, four rather distinguished areas should be covered, and

Table 5.3 Estimation of reliability (Cronbach's α) for the SRSS for German (GS3) and for English (ES1, ES2) samples and subsamples

				Cronbach's α			
		GS3	ES1	ES2			
				total	ANZ	UK	NA
	N	574	254	907	375	304	186
Short Recovery Scale		.70	.74	.84	.84	.81	.87
Short Stress Scale		.76	.78	.78	.76	.76	.83

Note: SRSS = *Short Recovery and Stress Scale*; ANZ = Australia/New Zealand; UK = United Kingdom; NA = North America

Table 5.4 Results of the internal consistency for the SRSS in the time course in study GS5 (N = 239)

	Items of the Short Recovery Scale				Items of the Short Stress Scale			
		α	M	SD		α	M	SD
T1	Physical Performance Capability	.72	4.46	1.06	Muscular Stress	.61	1.35	1.38
	Mental Performance Capability		4.69	0.93	Lack of Activation		0.46	0.85
	Emotional Balance		4.77	1.03	Negative Emotional State		0.70	0.98
	Overall Recovery		4.15	1.19	Overall Stress		1.16	1.14
T2	Physical Performance Capability	.71	4.76	0.92	Muscular Stress	.74	1.26	1.17
	Mental Performance Capability		4.92	1.01	Lack of Activation		0.46	0.83
	Emotional Balance		4.85	1.06	Negative Emotional State		0.53	0.87
	Overall Recovery		4.40	1.09	Overall Stress		1.02	1.16
T3	Physical Performance Capability	.74	3.58	1.26	Muscular Stress	.67	2.24	1.44
	Mental Performance Capability		4.25	1.22	Lack of Activation		0.84	1.17
	Emotional Balance		4.20	1.24	Negative Emotional State		0.98	1.12
	Overall Recovery		3.08	1.34	Overall Stress		2.18	1.41
T4	Physical Performance Capability	.76	4.36	1.06	Muscular Stress	.73	1.87	1.28
	Mental Performance Capability		4.81	0.94	Lack of Activation		0.67	1.04
	Emotional Balance		4.68	0.94	Negative Emotional State		0.59	0.84
	Overall Recovery		3.89	1.23	Overall Stress		1.69	1.25
T5	Physical Performance Capability	.73	3.59	1.20	Muscular Stress	.73	2.58	1.42
	Mental Performance Capability		4.35	1.22	Lack of Activation		0.98	1.30
	Emotional Balance		4.31	1.35	Negative Emotional State		1.03	1.31
	Overall Recovery		2.93	1.35	Overall Stress		2.58	1.59
T6	Physical Performance Capability	.78	4.08	1.07	Muscular Stress	.77	2.18	1.31
	Mental Performance Capability		4.70	1.02	Lack of Activation		0.88	1.19
	Emotional Balance		4.52	1.04	Negative Emotional State		0.91	1.14
	Overall Recovery		3.66	1.11	Overall Stress		2.18	1.40

Note: SRSS = *Short Recovery and Stress Scale*; T = Time of measurement; α = Internal consistency based on Cronbach's α

therefore the Cronbach's α does not necessarily have to be high for the *Short Recovery Scale* and the *Short Stress Scale*, while for the ARSS, each single scale should be high.

A similar scale homogeneity (α = .72) was found for the *Short Recovery Scale* in study GS5 for the first measurement. The *Short Stress Scale*, on the other hand, showed a lower value (α = .61) at the first time point of measurement for adolescents (Table 5.4).

However, an improved scale homogeneity could be observed over the duration of the study and especially for the measurements in the morning (T2, T4, T6). This suggests that participants become familiarized with the instrument and it can, hence, be recommended to use the instrument repeatedly.

Test-retest reliability

The SRSS is an instrument that focuses on the athlete's state, and no high test-retest reliability regarding the stability of measurements over time should be expected. Table 5.5 lists the correlations for the

Table 5.5 Spearman correlations (r_s) of the SRSS items for test-retest reliability for sample GS11

	Item	Day 1 (n = 51)	Day 1 & 2 (n = 53)	Day 1 & 8 (n = 53)	Day 1 & 26 (n = 50)
Short Recovery Scale	Physical Performance Capability	.46 [a]	.64 [a]	.38 [b]	.26 [d]
	Mental Performance Capability	.45 [a]	.53 [a]	.41 [b]	.49 [a]
	Emotional Balance	.48 [a]	.58 [a]	.33 [c]	.39 [b]
	Overall Recovery	.25 [d]	.37 [b]	.13 [d]	.32 [c]
Short Stress Scale	Muscular Stress	.43 [a]	.64 [a]	.51 [a]	.40 [b]
	Lack of Activation	.59 [a]	.53 [a]	.47 [a]	.36 [b]
	Negative Emotional State	.52 [a]	.63 [a]	.21 [d]	.29 [c]
	Overall Stress	.43 [b]	**.75** [a]	.47 [a]	.35 [c]

Note: SRSS = *Short Recovery and Stress Scale*; Day 1 = Beginning of the training camp and measurement in the evening; otherwise measurements in the morning

[a] = $p < .001$
[b] = $p < .01$
[c] = $p < .05$
[d] = non-significant; $r_s \geq .70$ are bolded

test-retest reliability for the duration of a four-week training camp in study GS11. The correlations were small, as expected, between the measurement in the morning and the measurement in the evening on day 1, as it was an intensive day with two training sessions. The comparatively highest correlations were measured between the first and the second morning, when the data were collected at the same time of day. The expected tendency of decreasing correlations was already evident after a week (between day 1 and day 8).

In study GS4, the German SRSS was used even more frequently (Hitzschke et al., 2015). The 25 field hockey players filled in the questionnaire three times per day: in the morning, in the evening, and they conducted an additional survey at lunchtime. When comparing morning and evening values, all recovery items showed a significant decrease in the evening on four days (*Mental Performance Capability* showed the decrease only on the first two days). The items of the *Short Stress Scale* increased significantly in the evening of the first two days only. The increase in the item *Lack of Activation* was even limited to day 1. In the course of the morning measurements, all items, except for *Lack of Activation* and *Negative Emotional State*, showed significant time effects. Across the evening measurements, all items stayed stable, except for *Physical Performance Capability* and *Overall Recovery*. Time effects were also found in the midday measurements for *Physical Performance Capability*, *Muscular Stress*, and *Overall Stress*.

These findings support the acute and sensitive recording of the athlete's recovery-stress state and a change in this state depending on training. The findings also support the test-retest reliability for short intervals at identical measurement times.

Construct validity

Construct validity has been studied with respect to the intercorrelations of the items and the stability of the intercorrelations across different samples. Relationships to mood states, Delayed-Onset Muscle Soreness, and other criteria are covered in the section on convergent and discriminant validity.

Item intercorrelations

The height of the item correlations proved to be stable across different samples; however, the fundamental correlation pattern was almost unchanged across all samples with respect to the *Short Recovery Scale* and the *Short Stress Scale*.

Based on the Spearman correlation coefficient, item intercorrelations within the short scales ranged from $r_s = .36$ to $r_s = .59$ for the *Short Recovery Scale* and from $r_s = .15$ to $r_s = 62$ for the *Short Stress Scale* for sample ES1. Correlations from $r_s = -.05$ to $r_s = -.66$ (Table 5.6) were measured between the items of the *Short Recovery Scale* and the *Short Stress Scale*.

Table 5.6 Spearman correlations (r_s) within the SRSS items for samples ES1 ($n = 254$) and ES2 ($n = 907$)

	Item	\multicolumn{8}{c}{Upper data matrix: ES2}
		PPC	MPC	EB	OR	MS	LA	NES	OS
Short Recovery Scale	Physical Performance Capability		.63 [a]	.52 [a]	.62 [a]	−.27 [a]	−.49 [a]	−.35 [a]	−.46 [a]
	Mental Performance Capability	.50 [a]		.66 [a]	.52 [a]	−.14 [a]	−.53 [a]	−.49 [a]	−.49 [a]
	Emotional Balance	.36 [a]	.58 [a]		.51 [a]	−.11 [a]	−.48 [a]	−.66 [a]	−.52 [a]
	Overall Recovery	.59 [a]	.47 [a]	.37 [a]		−.45 [a]	−.40 [a]	−.34 [a]	−.49 [a]
Short Stress Scale	Muscular Stress	−.26 [a]	−.11 [d]	−.05 [d]	−.45 [a]		.29 [a]	.21 [a]	.43 [a]
	Lack of Activation	−.36 [a]	−.39 [a]	−.51 [a]	−.41 [a]	.26 [a]		.63 [a]	.65 [a]
	Negative Emotional State	−.21 [c]	−.40 [a]	−.66 [a]	−.29 [a]	.15 [c]	.60 [a]		.64 [a]
	Overall Stress	−.35 [a]	−.38 [a]	−.48 [a]	−.50 [a]	.41 [a]	.62 [a]	.60 [a]	
		\multicolumn{8}{c}{Lower data matrix: ES1}

Note: SRSS = *Short Recovery and Stress Scale*; PPC = *Physical Performance Capability*; MPC = *Mental Performance Capability*; EB = *Emotional Balance*; OR = *Overall Recovery*; MS = *Muscular Stress*; LA = *Lack of Activation*; NES = *Negative Emotional State*; OS = *Overall Stress*; ES = English sample

[a] = $p < .001$
[b] = $p < .01$
[c] = $p < .05$
[d] = non-significant; lower data matrix modified from Nässi et al. (2017a)

Sample ES2 showed higher correlations within the dimensions, ranging from $r_s = .51$ to $r_s = .66$ for the *Short Recovery Scale* and from $r_s = .21$ to $r_s = .65$ for the *Short Stress Scale*. Correlations from $r_s = -.11$ to $r_s = -.66$ were found between the items of the *Short Recovery Scale* and the *Short Stress Scale* (Table 5.6). However, as seen in Table 5.7, the North American subsample consistently showed the highest item intercorrelations of the three subsamples (Australia/New Zealand, United Kingdom, North America).

The results are similar to that of the German ARSS, which showed item intercorrelations from $r_s = .46$ to $r_s = .71$ within the *Short Recovery Scale* and $r_s = .19$ to $r_s = .75$ within the *Short Stress Scale* (for sample GS3, see Appendix SRSS 2). Between the items of the *Short Recovery Scale* and the *Short Stress Scale*, correlations from $r_s = -.21$ to $r_s = -.71$ were observed.

Convergent and discriminant validity

The recovery-stress state was validated against a broad range of criteria, which covers psychological measures such as mood state, sensitivity to change, and performance, as well as physiological indicators.

Correlations with actual mood state

The expected relationships between the actual state and the SRSS have been empirically verified, which supports the validity of the SRSS. The relationship to the actual physical and psychological mood state has been covered by the correlations with the RESTQ-Sport-76, the DOMS, and the POMS.

RESTQ-Sport

Concurrent validity of the SRSS was assessed by examining the scores in relation to the RESTQ-Sport-76. All samples showed correlations with the scales of the RESTQ-Sport-76 that confirmed the hypothesis that positive correlations among the related RESTQ-Sport-76 scales/SRSS items and negative correlations between the opposite RESTQ-Sport-76 scales/SRSS items for both stress and recovery should occur (Kellmann et al., 2016).

Concurrent validity of the SRSS was shown for samples ES1 and ES2 (Table 5.8); a similar pattern but lower correlations were observed for the German SRSS (sample GS3; see Appendix SRSS 3). Positive correlations among the related scales/items and negative correlations between the opposite scales/items for both stress and recovery seemed to make up a clear pattern. For ES1/ES2, the English SRSS item *Physical Performance Capability* and the RESTQ-Sport-76 scale *Being in Shape* showed the strongest correlations

Table 5.7 Spearman correlations (r_s) within the SRSS items for subsamples ES2_ANZ ($n = 375$), ES2_UK ($n = 304$), and ES2_NA ($n = 186$)

	Item		PPC	MPC	EB	OR	MS	LA	NES	OS
Short Recovery Scale	Physical Performance Capability	ANZ		.61 [a]	.50 [a]	.60 [a]	−.25 [a]	−.46 [a]	−.33 [a]	−.44 [a]
		UK		.58 [a]	.44 [a]	.58 [a]	−.26 [a]	−.45 [a]	−.27 [a]	−.46 [a]
		NA		**.73** [a]	.64 [a]	.67 [a]	−.32 [a]	−.58 [a]	−.46 [a]	−.50 [a]
	Mental Performance Capability	ANZ			.66 [a]	.50 [a]	−.12 [c]	−.50 [a]	−.54 [a]	−.48 [a]
		UK			.60 [a]	.51 [a]	−.11 [d]	−.48 [a]	−.42 [a]	−.45 [a]
		NA			**.74** [a]	.55 [a]	−.20 [b]	−.60 [a]	−.53 [a]	−.54 [a]
	Emotional Balance	ANZ				.51 [a]	−.09 [d]	−.48 [a]	−.69 [a]	−.55 [a]
		UK				.48 [a]	−.11 [d]	−.45 [a]	−.66 [a]	−.42 [a]
		NA				.56 [a]	−.19 [c]	−.53 [a]	−.60 [a]	−.60 [a]
	Overall Recovery	ANZ					−.42 [a]	−.37 [a]	−.35 [a]	−.48 [a]
		UK					−.42 [a]	−.37 [a]	−.30 [a]	−.47 [a]
		NA					−.53 [a]	−.49 [a]	−.35 [a]	−.52 [a]
Short Stress Scale	Muscular Stress	ANZ						.24 [a]	.21 [a]	.42 [a]
		UK						.27 [a]	.16 [b]	.42 [a]
		NA						.42 [a]	.29 [a]	.51 [a]
	Lack of Activation	ANZ							.57 [a]	.58 [a]
		UK							.63 [a]	.68 [a]
		NA							**.72** [a]	**.73** [a]
	Negative Emotional State	ANZ								.66 [a]
		UK								.61 [a]
		NA								**.70** [a]
	Overall Stress	ANZ								
		UK								
		NA								

Note: SRSS = *Short Recovery and Stress Scale*; PPC = *Physical Performance Capability*; MPC = *Mental Performance Capability*; EB = *Emotional Balance*; OR = *Overall Recovery*; MS = *Muscular Stress*; LA = *Lack of Activation*; NES = *Negative Emotional State*; OS = *Overall Stress*; ES = English sample; ANZ = Australia/New Zealand; UK = United Kingdom; NA = North America

[a] = $p < .001$
[b] = $p < .01$
[c] = $p < .05$
[d] = non-significant; $r \geq .70$ are bolded

($r_s = .56 / .60$). *Muscular Stress* for the SRSS showed the highest correlation with the *Injury* RESTQ-Sport-76 scale ($r_s = .38 / .57$). *Negative Emotional State* (SRSS) and *General Stress* (RESTQ-Sport-76, $r_s = .60 / .68$) and *Emotional Stress* (RESTQ-Sport-76, $r_s = .60 / .65$) demonstrated noticeable correlations. In addition, *Emotional Balance* (SRSS) correlated clearly with *General Well-being* (RESTQ-Sport-76, $r_s = .55 / .65$) and *Overall Recovery* (SRSS) with *Physical Recovery* (RESTQ-Sport-76, $r_s = .44 / .51$).

The previously described pattern occurred for all three language regions: the Australian/New Zealand, United Kingdom, and North American subsamples (Table 5.9). However, the latter almost consistently showed the highest correlations.

DOMS

The highest correlations with the German DOMS were found with the item *Muscular Stress* ($r_s = .56$) in sample GS3 (Table 5.10), which highlights the construct validity of this item (see Hitzschke et al., 2016).

POMS

The original English version of the POMS is a 65-item Likert-format questionnaire with intensity scales ranging from '1' (*not at all*) to '4' (*extremely*). The POMS provides a measure of general mood disturbances

Table 5.8 Spearman correlations (r_s) of the SRSS items with the RESTQ-Sport-76 scales for samples ES1 (n = 254) and ES2 (n = 572)

ES1; ES2	RESTQ-Sport-76																		
	Overall Stress							Overall Recovery					Sport-specific Stress			Sport-specific Recovery			
	1	2	3	4	5	6	7	8	9	10	11	12	13	14	15	16	17	18	19
PPC	-.20 b	-.11 d	-.14 c	-.13 c	-.19 b	-.16 c	-.30 a	.27 a	.23 a	.46 a	.28 a	.21 b	-.12 d	-.15 c	-.22 a	.56 a	.30 a	.48 a	.28 a
	-.33 a	-.33 a	-.29 a	-.31 a	-.35 a	-.44 a	-.45 a	.42 a	.29 a	.54 a	.44 a	.28 a	-.24 a	-.30 a	-.36 a	.60 a	.36 a	.46 a	.38 a
MPC	-.35 a	-.28 a	-.31 a	-.15 c	-.23 a	-.22 a	-.31 a	.35 a	.18 b	.45 a	.43 a	.26 a	-.17 b	-.34 a	-.11 d	.45 a	.42 a	.44 a	.40 a
	-.49 a	-.46 a	-.38 a	-.40 a	-.41 a	-.55 a	-.46 a	.47 a	.33 a	.48 a	.49 a	.36 a	-.30 a	-.36 a	-.22 a	.49 a	.35 a	.46 a	.34 a
EB	-.59 a	-.50 a	-.48 a	-.38 a	-.29 a	-.42 a	-.39 a	.39 a	.36 a	.51 a	.55 a	.40 a	-.24 a	-.46 a	-.19 b	.47 a	.33 a	.44 a	.30 a
	-.63 a	-.57 a	-.47 a	-.48 a	-.40 a	-.52 a	-.48 a	.46 a	.38 a	.58 a	.65 a	.42 a	-.31 a	-.41 a	-.20 a	.49 a	.39 a	.45 a	.30 a
OR	-.30 a	-.21 b	-.28 a	-.22 b	-.31 a	-.20 b	-.37 a	.22 a	.16 c	.44 a	.31 a	.26 a	-.29 a	-.28 a	-.44 a	.44 a	.26 a	.32 a	.16 c
	-.29 a	-.30 a	-.22 a	-.36 a	-.41 a	-.36 a	-.45 a	.31 a	.20 a	.51 a	.37 a	.35 a	-.28 a	-.28 a	-.42 a	.49 a	.27 a	.34 a	.26 a
MS	.09 d	.09 d	.18 b	.09 d	.18 b	.10 d	.26 a	-.11 d	-.10 d	-.16 c	-.10 d	-.09 d	.19 b	.13 c	.38 a	-.19 b	-.17 b	-.08 d	.00 d
	.13 a	.17 a	.16 a	.22 a	.32 a	.23 a	.38 a	-.16 a	-.03 d	-.25 a	-.09 c	-.18 a	.27 a	.23 a	.57 a	-.25 a	-.07 d	-.11 b	-.06 d
LA	.51 a	.48 a	.43 a	.34 a	.44 a	.48 a	.45 a	-.39 a	-.27 a	-.46 a	-.46 a	-.45 a	.38 a	.49 a	.29 a	-.48 a	-.33 a	-.40 a	-.29 b
	.53 a	.49 a	.44 a	.41 a	.43 a	.59 a	.54 a	-.42 a	-.27 a	-.49 a	-.47 a	-.36 a	.36 a	.49 a	.32 a	-.51 a	-.30 a	-.44 a	-.36 a
NES	.60 a	.60 a	.53 a	.44 a	.35 a	.47 a	.37 a	-.32 a	-.29 a	-.45 a	-.52 a	-.37 a	.27 a	.50 a	.20 b	-.39 a	-.35 a	-.32 a	-.27 b
	.68 a	.65 a	.58 a	.52 a	.42 a	.52 a	.55 a	-.40 a	-.40 a	-.54 a	-.61 a	-.43 a	.35 a	.50 a	.24 a	-.48 a	-.36 a	-.45 a	-.29 a
OS	.46 a	.44 a	.46 a	.38 a	.46 a	.42 a	.47 a	-.31 a	-.16 b	-.45 a	-.38 a	-.41 a	.38 a	.46 a	.33 a	-.37 a	-.31 a	-.30 a	-.18 b
	.53 a	.53 a	.44 a	.51 a	.55 a	.53 a	.58 a	-.31 a	-.25 a	-.51 a	-.43 a	-.43 a	.41 a	.47 a	.38 a	-.48 a	-.28 a	-.39 a	-.26 a

Note: a = $p < .001$
b = $p < .01$
c = $p < .05$
d = non-significant; ES = English sample

SRSS = Short Recovery and Stress Scale; PPC = Physical Performance Capability; MPC = Mental Performance Capability; EB = Emotional Balance; OR = Overall Recovery; MS = Muscular Stress; LA = Lack of Activation; NES = Negative Emotional State; OS = Overall Stress; RESTQ-Sport-76 = Recovery-Stress Questionnaire for Athletes; RESTQ-Sport-76 scales: 1 = General Stress; 2 = Emotional Stress; 3 = Social Stress; 4 = Conflicts/Pressure; 5 = Fatigue; 6 = Lack of Energy; 7 = Physical Complaints; 8 = Success; 9 = Social Recovery; 10 = Physical Recovery; 11 = General Well-being; 12 = Sleep Quality; 13 = Disturbed Breaks; 14 = Emotional Exhaustion; 15 = Injury; 16 = Being in Shape; 17 = Personal Accomplishment; 18 = Self-Efficacy; 19 = Self-Regulation

Table 5.9 Spearman correlations (r_s) of the SRSS items with the RESTQ_Sport-76 scales for the subsamples ES2_ANZ ($n = 239$), ES2_UK ($n = 126$), and ES2_NA ($n = 165$)

		RESTQ-Sport-76																		
		Overall Stress							Overall Recovery					Sport-specific Stress			Sport-specific Recovery			
		1	2	3	4	5	6	7	8	9	10	11	12	13	14	15	16	17	18	19
PPC	ANZ	-.27 [a]	-.27 [a]	-.23 [a]	-.28 [a]	-.29 [a]	-.42 [a]	-.43 [a]	.30 [a]	.25 [a]	.47 [a]	.36 [a]	.27 [a]	-.21 [a]	-.24 [a]	-.35 [a]	.49 [a]	.27 [a]	.30 [a]	.23 [a]
	UK	-.31 [a]	-.33 [a]	-.28 [b]	-.31 [a]	-.38 [a]	-.49 [a]	-.37 [a]	.43 [a]	.19 [c]	.49 [a]	.38 [a]	.22 [c]	-.21 [c]	-.27 [b]	-.31 [a]	.63 [a]	.34 [a]	.52 [a]	.39 [a]
	NA	-.44 [a]	-.43 [a]	-.36 [a]	-.36 [a]	-.38 [a]	-.46 [a]	-.54 [a]	.52 [a]	.43 [a]	.66 [a]	.61 [a]	.36 [a]	-.28 [a]	-.41 [a]	-.41 [a]	.71 [a]	.45 [a]	.59 [a]	.49 [a]
MPC	ANZ	-.50 [a]	-.39 [a]	-.35 [a]	-.38 [a]	-.35 [a]	-.54 [a]	-.42 [a]	.44 [a]	.34 [a]	.52 [a]	.50 [a]	.36 [a]	-.28 [a]	-.36 [a]	-.18 [b]	.43 [a]	.31 [a]	.41 [a]	.28 [a]
	UK	-.45 [a]	-.47 [a]	-.40 [a]	-.34 [a]	-.36 [a]	-.52 [a]	-.37 [a]	.46 [a]	.29 [a]	.36 [a]	.44 [a]	.27 [b]	-.14 [d]	-.33 [a]	-.14 [d]	.41 [a]	.27 [b]	.38 [a]	.26 [b]
	NA	-.56 [a]	-.61 [a]	-.47 [a]	-.46 [a]	-.47 [a]	-.61 [a]	-.56 [a]	.50 [a]	.38 [a]	.55 [a]	.55 [a]	.45 [a]	-.39 [a]	-.45 [a]	-.27 [a]	.64 [a]	.47 [a]	.59 [a]	.44 [a]
EB	ANZ	-.63 [a]	-.54 [a]	-.44 [a]	-.47 [a]	-.37 [a]	-.49 [a]	-.45 [a]	.38 [a]	.39 [a]	.58 [a]	.62 [a]	.41 [a]	-.33 [a]	-.46 [a]	-.21 [b]	.41 [a]	.36 [a]	.38 [a]	.17 [b]
	UK	-.61 [a]	-.54 [a]	-.42 [a]	-.42 [a]	-.35 [a]	-.56 [a]	-.41 [a]	.56 [a]	.25 [b]	.60 [a]	.66 [a]	.40 [a]	-.09 [c]	-.23 [c]	-.09 [d]	.44 [a]	.29 [a]	.42 [a]	.32 [a]
	NA	-.61 [a]	-.63 [a]	-.51 [a]	-.53 [a]	-.44 [a]	-.53 [a]	-.51 [a]	.47 [a]	.47 [a]	.59 [a]	.68 [a]	.44 [a]	-.34 [a]	-.47 [a]	-.26 [a]	.64 [a]	.45 [a]	.54 [a]	.37 [a]
OR	ANZ	-.28 [a]	-.30 [a]	-.26 [a]	-.39 [a]	-.37 [a]	-.37 [a]	-.42 [a]	.21 [a]	.21 [a]	.40 [a]	.36 [a]	.36 [a]	-.27 [a]	-.28 [a]	-.41 [a]	.37 [a]	.23 [a]	.22 [a]	.12 [d]
	UK	-.31 [a]	-.26 [b]	-.21 [c]	-.33 [a]	-.42 [a]	-.41 [a]	-.44 [a]	.35 [a]	.13 [d]	.45 [a]	.32 [a]	.30 [a]	-.27 [b]	-.24 [b]	-.32 [a]	.50 [a]	.10 [d]	.41 [a]	.26 [b]
	NA	-.29 [a]	-.33 [a]	-.24 [b]	-.32 [a]	-.40 [a]	-.35 [a]	-.51 [a]	.37 [a]	.23 [b]	.65 [a]	.45 [a]	.33 [a]	-.27 [a]	-.32 [a]	-.52 [a]	.61 [a]	.40 [a]	.44 [a]	.36 [a]
MS	ANZ	.13 [c]	.21 [a]	.21 [a]	.26 [a]	.39 [a]	.24 [a]	.35 [a]	-.09 [d]	-.02 [d]	-.16 [a]	-.05 [d]	-.20 [b]	.27 [a]	.24 [a]	.55 [a]	-.20 [b]	-.03 [d]	-.01 [d]	.01 [d]
	UK	.13 [d]	.13 [d]	.14 [d]	.16 [d]	.21 [c]	.21 [c]	.37 [a]	-.20 [c]	-.05 [d]	-.28 [a]	-.07 [d]	-.13 [d]	.19 [c]	.13 [d]	.55 [a]	-.27 [b]	.05 [d]	-.20 [c]	-.08 [d]
	NA	.16 [c]	.19 [c]	.15 [d]	.26 [a]	.34 [a]	.27 [a]	.47 [a]	-.21 [b]	-.11 [d]	-.36 [a]	-.18 [c]	-.23 [b]	.33 [a]	.29 [a]	.62 [a]	-.34 [a]	-.20 [b]	-.23 [b]	-.14 [d]
LA	ANZ	.47 [a]	.36 [a]	.36 [a]	.32 [a]	.37 [a]	.57 [a]	.48 [a]	-.41 [a]	-.27 [a]	-.49 [a]	-.45 [a]	-.31 [a]	.31 [a]	.47 [a]	.23 [a]	-.47 [a]	-.33 [a]	-.37 [a]	-.28 [a]
	UK	.62 [a]	.59 [a]	.54 [a]	.47 [a]	.42 [a]	.62 [a]	.49 [a]	-.43 [a]	-.24 [b]	-.49 [a]	-.48 [a]	-.37 [a]	.25 [b]	.50 [a]	.29 [a]	-.52 [a]	-.16 [d]	-.49 [a]	-.38 [a]
	NA	.57 [a]	.57 [a]	.49 [a]	.46 [a]	.46 [a]	.57 [a]	.62 [a]	-.37 [a]	-.31 [a]	-.56 [a]	-.52 [a]	-.47 [a]	.44 [a]	.54 [a]	.38 [a]	-.60 [a]	-.34 [a]	-.49 [a]	-.43 [a]
NES	ANZ	.68 [a]	.63 [a]	.59 [a]	.54 [a]	.38 [a]	.55 [a]	.55 [a]	-.42 [a]	-.42 [a]	-.58 [a]	-.63 [a]	-.50 [a]	.38 [a]	.58 [a]	.21 [a]	-.50 [a]	-.42 [a]	-.48 [a]	-.26 [a]
	UK	.71 [a]	.66 [a]	.60 [a]	.47 [a]	.38 [a]	.53 [a]	.44 [a]	-.42 [a]	-.34 [a]	-.47 [a]	-.58 [a]	-.29 [a]	.19 [c]	.45 [a]	.13 [d]	-.40 [a]	-.18 [c]	-.36 [a]	-.26 [b]
	NA	.68 [a]	.69 [a]	.61 [a]	.53 [a]	.48 [a]	.53 [a]	.63 [a]	-.37 [a]	-.47 [a]	-.59 [a]	-.63 [a]	-.48 [a]	.38 [a]	.50 [a]	.34 [a]	-.58 [a]	-.45 [a]	-.48 [a]	-.34 [a]
OS	ANZ	.50 [a]	.48 [a]	.44 [a]	.50 [a]	.50 [a]	.53 [a]	.49 [a]	-.26 [a]	-.26 [a]	-.44 [a]	-.42 [a]	-.44 [a]	.36 [a]	.48 [a]	.34 [a]	-.41 [a]	-.27 [a]	-.35 [a]	-.21 [a]
	UK	.52 [a]	.47 [a]	.43 [a]	.40 [a]	.45 [a]	.49 [a]	.57 [a]	-.34 [a]	-.17 [d]	-.42 [a]	-.33 [a]	-.30 [a]	.31 [a]	.43 [a]	.35 [a]	-.50 [a]	-.09 [d]	-.38 [a]	-.18 [c]
	NA	.55 [a]	.61 [a]	.47 [a]	.56 [a]	.60 [a]	.58 [a]	.66 [a]	-.33 [a]	-.30 [a]	-.63 [a]	-.50 [a]	-.48 [a]	.48 [a]	.54 [a]	.44 [a]	-.57 [a]	-.38 [a]	-.46 [a]	-.32 [a]

Note: [a] = $p < .001$
[b] = $p < .01$
[c] = $p < .05$
[d] = non-significant; $r \geq .70$ are bolded

ES = English sample; ANZ = Australia/New Zealand; UK = United Kingdom; NA = North America

SRSS = Short Recovery and Stress Scale; PPC = Physical Performance Capability; MPC = Mental Performance Capability; EB = Emotional Balance; OR = Overall Recovery; MS = Muscular Stress; LA = Lack of Activation; NES = Negative Emotional State; OS = Overall Stress; RESTQ-Sport-76 = Recovery-Stress Questionnaire for Athletes; RESTQ-Sport-76 scales: 1 = General Stress; 2 = Emotional Stress; 3 = Social Stress; 4 = Conflicts/Pressure; 5 = Fatigue; 6 = Lack of Energy; 7 = Physical Complaints; 8 = Success; 9 = Social Recovery; 10 = Physical Recovery; 11 = General Well-being; 12 = Sleep Quality; 13 = Disturbed Breaks; 14 = Emotional Exhaustion; 15 = Injury; 16 = Being in Shape; 17 = Personal Accomplishment; 18 = Self-Efficacy; 19 = Self-Regulation and six mood states (*Tension, Depression, Anger, Vigor, Fatigue, Confusion*). The same time frame ('right now') was used for the SRSS and POMS. Although the SRSS and the POMS apply different types of scales (frequency vs. intensity; Diener & Emmons, 1984), analysis revealed close and theoretically expected correlation patterns.

Tension, Depression, Anger, Fatigue, and *Confusion* negatively correlated with recovery-related items, whereas for *Vigor*, a positive relationship occurred (Table 5.10). The stress-related SRSS items showed positive correlations with *Tension, Depression, Anger, Fatigue,* and *Confusion,* but a negative correlation was found with *Vigor* for sample ES2. An analysis across two English language regions revealed a similar correlation pattern (*Muscular Stress* and *Vigor* showed opposite signs for the subsamples) for the Australian/New Zealand and United Kingdom subsamples of ES2 (Table 5.11).

Sensitivity to change

Due to the concise and economical design of the SRSS, one essential condition for the validity of the questionnaire is the sensitive recording of changes, which has to be seen in the context of the respective situation and is dependent on stress and recovery stimuli. Another condition is the assessment of the current recovery-stress state. There are laboratory studies (studies GS8–GS10) and field studies (studies GS11 and GS12) that have recorded this change.

Laboratory studies

STRENGTH TRAINING

Similar to the design of study GS6, 23 male and female athletes,[3] who were experienced in strength training, completed an intensive six-day strength training in sample GS8 (Raeder et al., 2016). The SRSS data, which were logged in the morning, were compared during a nine-day period (including four post-measurements). The item *Physical Performance Capability* already showed a significant decrease after the first training day and was still reduced in the second post-measurement. From pre- to the first post-measurement, the value decreased from 4.0 ± 1.0 to 2.4 ± 1.2. Only the fourth post-measurement showed the initial value from the beginning of the training period ($M = 4.0 \pm 1.3$). Similar results were found for the values of the item *Muscular Stress*, which increased from the second morning onwards and was significantly higher until the second post-measurement. The initial value of 1.6 ± 1.0 increased in the second post-measurement (3.9 ± 1.3) and decreased in the post-measurement (1.4 ± 1.2).

Table 5.10 Spearman correlations (r_s) between the DOMS and the SRSS for sample GS3 ($N = 574$), as well as the POMS and the SRSS for the sample ES2 ($n = 114$)

	Item	DOMS	POMS						
			Tension	Depression	Anger	Vigor	Fatigue	Confusion	TMD
Short Recovery Scale	Physical Performance Capability	−.27 [a]	−.42 [a]	−.35 [a]	−.31 [a]	.56 [a]	−.42 [a]	−.33 [a]	−.47 [a]
	Mental Performance Capability	−.17 [a]	−.59 [a]	−.51 [a]	−.40 [a]	.61 [a]	−.50 [a]	−.57 [a]	−.63 [a]
	Emotional Balance	−.08 [a]	−.63 [a]	−.54 [a]	−.47 [a]	.56 [a]	−.50 [a]	−.57 [a]	−.64 [a]
	Overall Recovery	−.36 [a]	−.44 [a]	−.37 [a]	−.35 [a]	.53 [a]	−.50 [a]	−.40 [a]	−.51 [a]
Short Stress Scale	Muscular Stress	.56 [a]	.20 [c]	.05 [d]	.10 [d]	−.12 [d]	.18 [d]	.11 [d]	.16 [d]
	Lack of Activation	.09 [a]	.62 [a]	.57 [a]	.49 [a]	−.64 [a]	.59 [a]	.56 [a]	.67 [a]
	Negative Emotional State	.11 [a]	**.73** [a]	.63 [a]	.64 [a]	−.55 [a]	.60 [a]	.61 [a]	**.74** [a]
	Overall Stress	.42 [a]	**.70** [a]	.60 [a]	.60 [a]	−.54 [a]	.69 [a]	.55 [a]	**.73** [a]

Note: SRSS = *Short Recovery and Stress Scale*; DOMS = Delayed-Onset Muscle Soreness; TMD = Total Mood Disturbance; GS = German sample; ES = English sample

[a] = $p < .001$
[b] = $p < .01$
[c] = $p < .05$
[d] = non-significant; $r_s \geq .70$ are bolded

Table 5.11 Spearman correlations (r_s) between the POMS and the SRSS for the subsamples ES2_ANZ (top line, $n = 61$) and ES2_UK (bottom line, $n = 42$)

	Item	POMS						
		Tension	Depression	Anger	Vigor	Fatigue	Confusion	TMD
Short Recovery Scale	Physical Performance Capability	−.43 [a] −.20 [d]	−.31 [c] −.21 [d]	−.24 [d] −.20 [d]	.50 [a] .54 [a]	−.44 [a] −.23 [d]	−.30 [c] −.18 [d]	−.49 [a] −.29 [d]
	Mental Performance Capability	−.58 [a] −.36 [c]	−.53 [a] −.27 [d]	−.35 [b] −.27 [d]	.56 [a] .57 [a]	−.48 [a] −.32 [c]	−.50 [a] −.48 [a]	−.61 [a] −.43 [b]
	Emotional Balance	−.59 [a] −.50 [a]	−.52 [a] −.41 [b]	−.41 [a] −.40 [b]	.45 [a] .57 [a]	−.45 [a] −.35 [c]	−.49 [a] −.53 [a]	−.59 [a] −.54 [a]
	Overall Recovery	−.47 [a] −.17 [d]	−.42 [a] −.16 [d]	−.32 [c] −.23 [d]	.53 [a] .39 [c]	−.52 [a] −.35 [c]	−.34 [b] −.29 [d]	−.56 [a] −.29 [d]
Short Stress Scale	Muscular Stress	.20 [d] .23 [d]	.02 [d] .10 [d]	.01 [d] .11 [d]	−.19 [d] .10 [d]	.29 [c] .01 [d]	.08 [d] .01 [d]	.17 [d] .09 [d]
	Lack of Activation	.56 [a] .54 [a]	.53 [a] .49 [a]	.40 [a] .50 [a]	−.61 [a] −.52 [a]	.53 [a] .54 [a]	.53 [a] .52 [a]	.64 [a] .59 [a]
	Negative Emotional State	.68 [a] .65 [a]	.62 [a] .61 [a]	.58 [a] .68 [a]	−.49 [a] −.42 [b]	.53 [a] .62 [a]	.54 [a] **.71** [a]	.69 [a] **.73** [a]
	Overall Stress	.64 [a] .58 [a]	.55 [a] .52 [a]	.50 [a] .59 [a]	−.54 [a] −.27 [a]	.66 [a] .56 [a]	.48 [a] .51 [a]	**.70** [a] .61 [a]

Note: SRSS = *Short Recovery and Stress Scale*; POMS = Profile of Mood States; TMD = Total Mood Disturbance; ES = English sample; ANZ = Australia/New Zealand; UK = United Kingdom

[a] = $p < .001$
[b] = $p < .01$
[c] = $p < .05$
[d] = non-significant; $r_s \geq .70$ are bolded

TENNIS

Another intervention study (sample GS9) compared active and passive recovery for a four-day high-intensity interval training (HIIT) with eight adolescent top tennis players (Wiewelhove et al., 2016). During the four weeks between training camps, the athletes used active and passive recovery strategies after each training session. The SRSS was filled in one day before and one day after the shock microcycles. All eight items showed a significant time effect that was independent from the intervention. Except for the item *Emotional Balance*, all recovery values decreased with high to very high effect sizes from pre- to post-measurements when recovering passively. The clearest difference could be seen in *Overall Recovery*, with the largest decrease when recovering passively ($M = 4.9 \pm 1.0$ to $M = 2.5 \pm 0.9$). Equally, all items of the *Short Stress Scale* showed significant increases in the post-measurement. *Muscular Stress* increased the most with both passive ($M = 0.8 \pm 0.7$ to $M = 3.8 \pm 1.1$) and active ($M = 0.5 \pm 0.8$ to $M = 3.5 \pm 1.7$) recovery strategies. While large to very large effect sizes were found for the physical and general recovery and stress items, only small to medium effect sizes were measured for the emotional and mental items. This emphasizes the rather physically demanding nature of the training protocol (Wiewelhove et al., 2016).

PSYCHOLOGICAL RECOVERY STRATEGIES

The sensitivity to change on *Overall Recovery* was especially visible in the experimental study GS10. The SRSS was completed four times within approximately 90 minutes (Pelka, Kölling, et al., 2017). The aim of the study was to test the effect of different recovery strategies (breathing regulation, yoga, progressive muscle relaxation, power napping) on the sprinting performance of the 27 female and male participants. The short 25-minute recovery session was embedded in between two repeated sprint tests. The SRSS was completed under resting conditions before sprinting, after the first sprint test, after the recovery break, and after the last sprint test. Independent of the content of the intervention condition, the item *Overall*

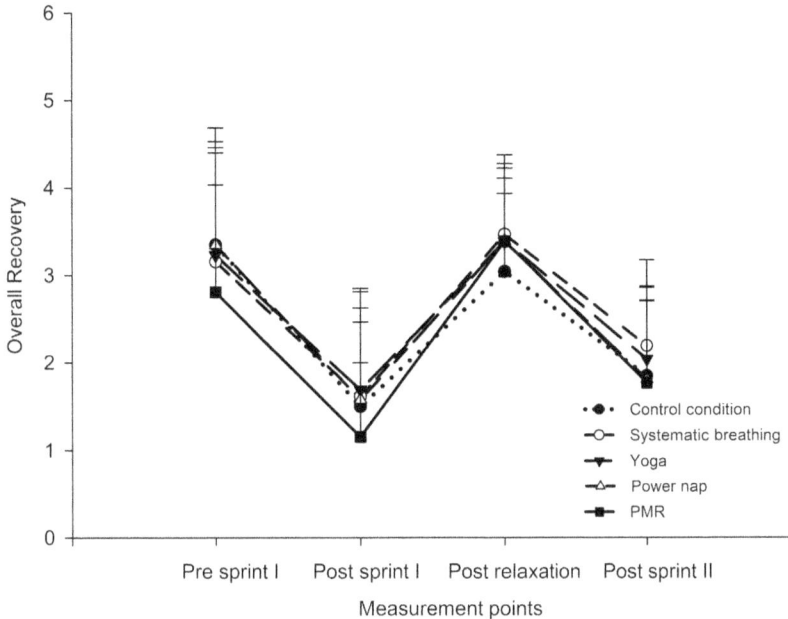

Figure 5.2 Development of the *Overall Recovery* states over the course of an experimental day
Source: reprinted, with permission, from Pelka, Kölling, et al., 2017, p. 220

Recovery (as expected) showed a 'zigzag-shaped' development matching the course of the intervention (Figure 5.2).

A clear decrease in *Overall Recovery* could be seen after the first sprint, while after the recovery break the initial level was roughly reclaimed. Interestingly, the value for *Overall Recovery* decreased after the second sprint, as well. However, the value did not drop to the same level as after the first sprint. Consequently, the SRSS helped to show that even a short observation period can record variability in the state of recovery after physical stress.

Field studies

ROWING

In a field study (study GS11), Kölling et al. (2016) monitored athletes in a four-week training camp of the German national U19 rowing team. The monitoring was done during the team's preparation for the immediately following World Rowing Junior Championship. Every morning, 30 male and 25 female rowers filled in a sleep log (based on Hoffmann, Müller, Hajak, & Cassel, 1997) and the SRSS. The SRSS data showed very little variability for the whole training group during the first three weeks over the 26 days of measurement (Figure 5.3).

This was especially true for the items *Emotional Balance* and *Negative Emotional State*, as well as for *Mental Performance Capability* and *Lack of Activation*, which showed the lowest variability in the first three weeks. However, this development highlights even more the effect of the only training-free day (day 22). There was no training scheduled, and the athletes could sleep in. Every single item of the *Short Recovery Scale* showed peak values on this day. The items of the *Short Stress Scale*, on the other hand, showed their lowest values. The physical, muscular, and general recovery items in particular continued at an elevated level, whereas the stress items decreased respectively. In addition, an analysis of the comparison with the day before and the day after proved that all values of the *Short Recovery Scale* increased significantly, and all values of the *Short Stress Scale* decreased significantly.

Furthermore, the training camp showed a correlation between the SRSS and the athletes' sleep behavior (Kölling et al., 2016). To determine this pattern, the first six days were summarized to form a baseline. These values were then correlated with information from the sleep log. A sleep that is perceived as restful

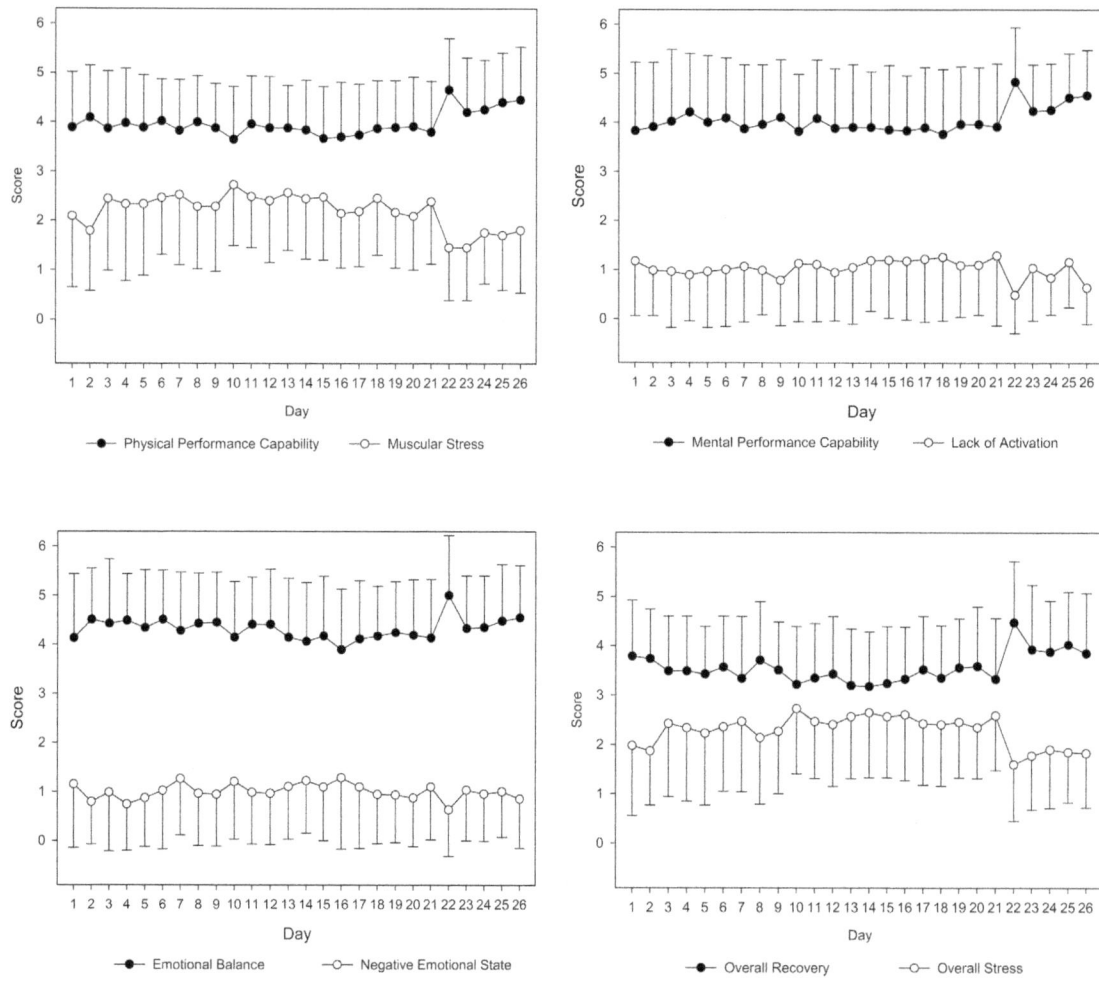

Figure 5.3 Overview of the *Short Recovery and Stress Scale* ratings over 26 days for sample GS11

Source: reprinted, with permission, from Kölling et al., 2016, p. 78

(on a scale from '1' = *very* to '5' = *not at all*) correlated with a high rating in the item *Physical Performance Capability* ($r = -.29$) and a high value in *Overall Recovery* ($r = -.28$). A correlation was also found between frequent waking up at night and a low value on the *Overall Recovery* item the next morning ($r = -.28$).

Moreover, changes in the SRSS values in relation to sleep duration could be observed. During the football World Cup final in July 2014 (Germany vs. Argentina), the average night's bedtime changed from 10 p.m. to 11:30 p.m., while the training session the next day (day 7) started at 6:30 a.m. as usual. Due to the shorter sleeping time, the value on the item *Overall Recovery* decreased temporarily. The value on the item *Negative Emotional State* was higher due to the shorter sleeping time, but it decreased again the next morning (Kölling et al., 2016).

FOOTBALL

The aim of the study GS12 by Pelka et al. (2018) was to examine how competitive matches affect self-report measures of physical, mental, and emotional states. A total of 25 players ($M = 17.5 \pm 0.5$ years) of an U19 junior Bundesliga team (highest German football league for this particular age group) participated over the entire six-month assessment period. The players completed the SRSS twice a week on Monday and Friday mornings between 7 a.m. and 9 a.m. During the assessment period, the players participated in 12 match days. Wilcoxon signed-rank tests revealed significant main effects for

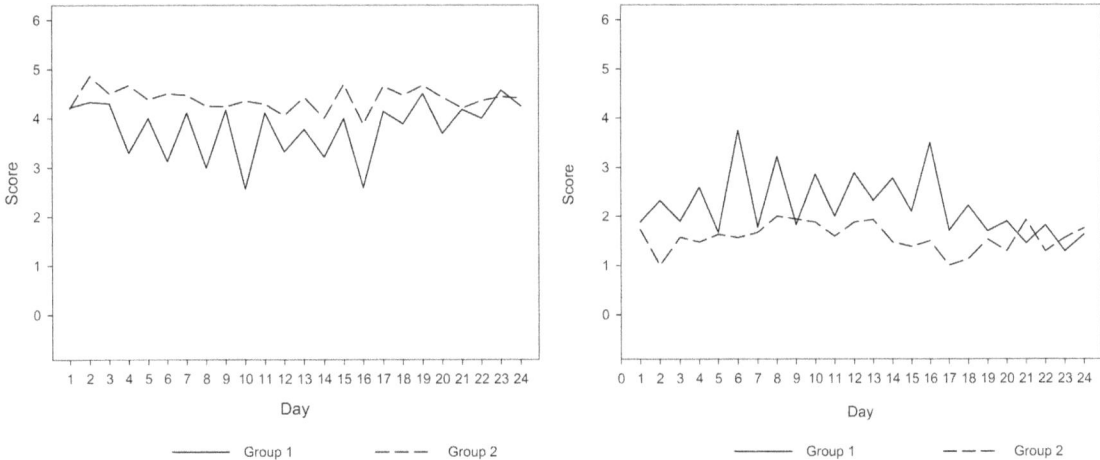

Figure 5.4 Seasonal change and variation in *Physical Performance Capability* [left] and *Muscular Stress* [right] ratings

Note: The solid and the dotted line represent the respective group means on the 24 test days (Mondays = even numbers, Fridays = uneven numbers) over the course of the 12 matches, which were considered for the analysis. Group 1 = players who played more than 60 minutes; Group 2 = players who played less than 60 minutes

Source: reprinted, with permission, from Pelka et al., 2018, p. 130

changes in *Physical Performance Capability* and *Muscular Stress* from Friday to Monday ratings in players who played more than 60 minutes (group 1) and less than 60 minutes (group 2; see Figure 5.4).

The regular players were more physically and mentally stressed after matches, whereas the substitutes experienced higher emotional stress when comparing Mondays' and Fridays' stress ratings. Therefore, matches affected those who played more than 60 minutes differently compared with those who played less than 60 minutes. This was not only the case for physical recovery-stress ratings, but also for mental, emotional, and overall self-reports.

Performance parameters

Hitzschke et al. (2017) aimed at investigating the effect of intensive microcycles in strength and high-intensity interval training on subjective measures of recovery and stress, and to descriptively compare these effects with variations among performance parameters. It was shown that the subjective perspective, measured via the SRSS items, reflected fatigue and recovery phases in a very sensitive and practical way, but could not exactly differentiate between athletes in fatigued or recovered states in relation to performance criterion measures. However, similar to the results of the ARSS (Figure 4.8), the descriptive data of SRSS items and the counter movement jump, as presented in Figure 5.5, indicated a correspondence of subjective and objective parameters.

Physiological response

Creatine kinase

Creatine kinase (CK) was chosen as a physiological parameter to assess information about muscle damage due to training. Several studies have tracked CK during training and competition as a marker of muscle damage or increased membrane permeability to the enzyme (Meeusen et al., 2013). Serum CK activity usually increases in response to strength training, especially due to eccentric exercise (Hortobagyi & Denahan, 1989) and normalizes when muscular adaptation occurs with training (Steinacker et al., 1998).

Two experimental studies, by Wiewelhove et al. (2015) and Raeder et al. (2016), were designed to induce functional overload in athletes by having them train at their individual maximal tolerable capacity. In total, 11 training sessions were completed (i.e., two sessions per day except for day 5; for a detailed overview, see Figure 6.1). During the experimental period, participants were instructed to maintain their normal dietary intake, which was recorded via food diaries, and habitual lifestyle while refraining from alcohol.

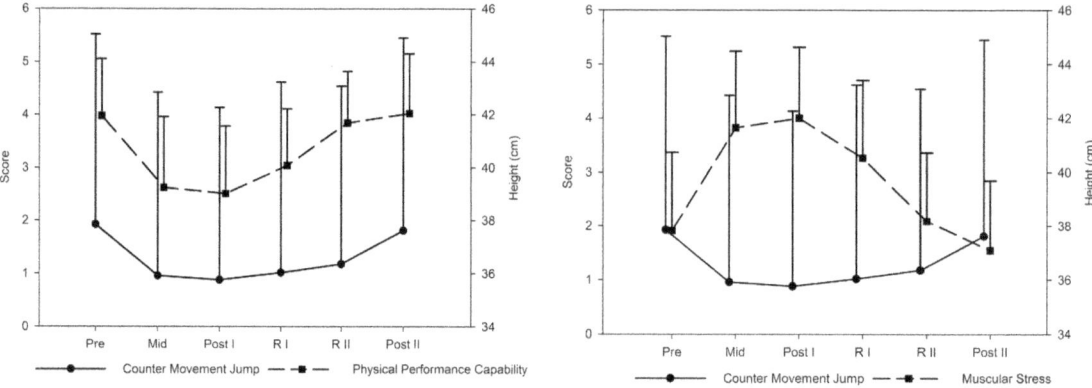

Figure 5.5 Changes of counter movement jump and the SRSS items *Physical Performance Capability* [left] and *Muscular Stress* [right] during the study

Note: Pre = Pre-test; Mid = Mid-test; Post = Post-test; R = Recovery; SRSS = *Short Recovery and Stress Scale*

Source: unpublished data from Wiewelhove et al., 2015; Raeder et al., 2016

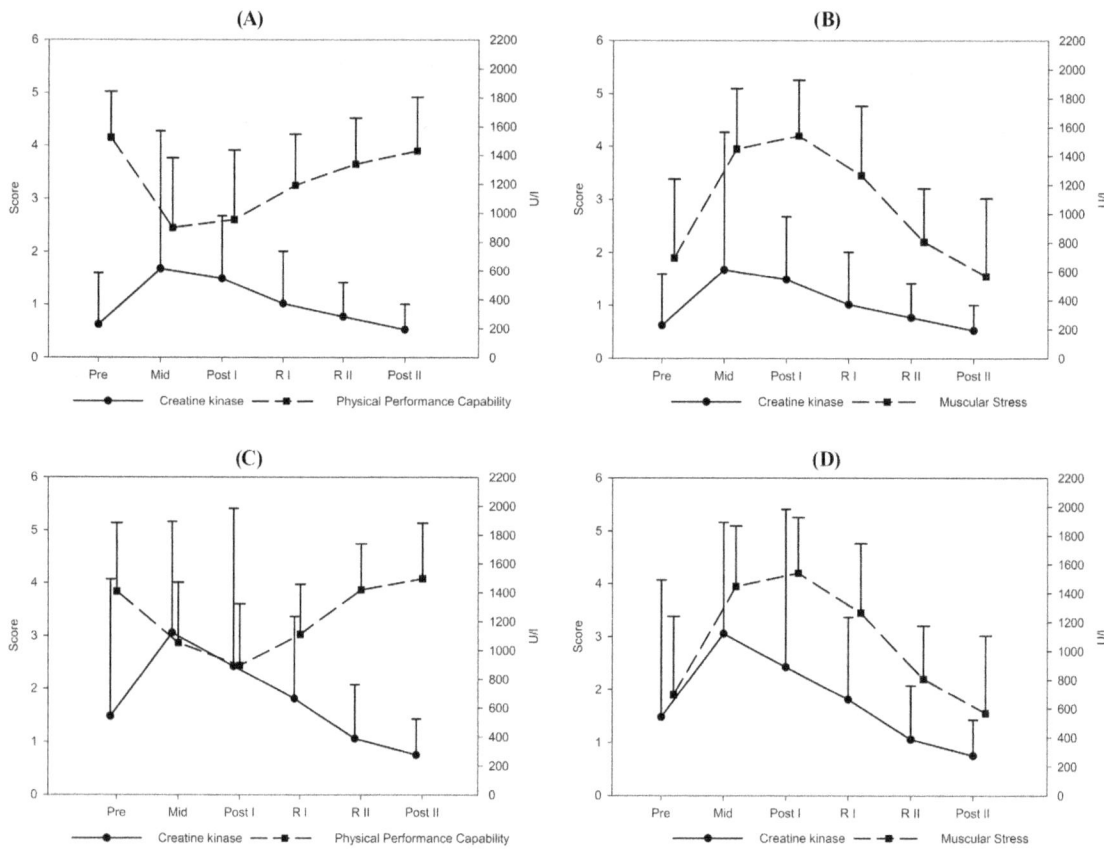

Figure 5.6 Changes of Creatine kinase (U/l) and the SRSS items *Physical Performance Capability* [A] and *Muscular Stress* [B] for females and *Physical Performance Capability* [C] and *Muscular Stress* [D] for males

Note: Pre = Pre-test; Mid = Mid-test; Post = Post-test; R = Recovery; SRSS = *Short Recovery and Stress Scale*

Source: unpublished data from Wiewelhove et al., 2015; Raeder et al., 2016

No irregular dietary habits were observed, which was crucial for comparable conditions on testing days. Throughout the five baseline days and the three-day post assessment, participants were asked to refrain from intensive training or excessive physical activity. Moreover, participants did not apply systematic recovery strategies for the entire period.

Similar to the ARSS results (Figure 4.6), the muscle damage due to training and its physical indicator CK were mirrored by the subjective rating of *Muscular Stress* and inversely related to *Physical Performance Capability* (Figure 5.6) of the SRSS.

The present results suggest that a dose-response relationship exists between training load, CK, and the subjective assessment of stress and recovery. A high training load is indicated by elevated levels of stress and simultaneous lowered levels of recovery, which is supported by findings from Kellmann et al. (2001) and those by Kellmann and Günther (2000).

Summary of the SRSS

The SRSS assesses the current recovery-stress state of an athlete on emotional, mental, physical, and overall levels. The SRSS is a standardized self-assessment procedure and includes the items *Physical Performance Capability*, *Mental Performance Capability*, *Emotional Balance*, and *Overall Recovery* in the *Short Recovery Scale*; and *Muscular Stress*, *Lack of Activation*, *Negative Emotional State*, and *Overall Stress* in the *Short Stress Scale*. The SRSS was derived from the eight scales of the ARSS, which were then grouped into the *Short Recovery Scale* and the *Short Stress Scale* and consists of four items each. As descriptors the adjectives from the ARSS are listed underneath the SRSS items for a better understanding only. The level of agreement is determined by a seven-point Likert scale ('0' = *does not apply at all* to '6' = *fully applies*). The SRSS is a reliable and valid instrument. Cronbach's α for ES2 ($N = 907$) ranges between $\alpha = .78$ and $\alpha = .84$. The convergent and construct validity is supported through theory-conform relationships with the established instruments RESTQ-Sport-76, POMS, and DOMS in sport-specific stress and rest situations. The sensitivity to change could also be verified in the training monitoring of different sports which, however, still needs to be confirmed for the English version. The SRSS is economical and especially useful for high-frequency use (e.g., in the daily monitoring of training). Completion time for the SRSS ranges between 40 and 60 seconds.

Notes

1 Recent data of the German SRSS for a sample of children (10–13 years, $n = 312$) indicate that an explanatory sentence for each item leads to a better understanding. A similar effect occurs also for the age group 14–16 years (with additional explanation, $n = 441$; without explanation, $n = 303$). By the end of 2018, there are no substantial samples/data from children and adolescents available for the English version to support similar conclusions.
2 Please note: We strongly emphasize that the instruction, the order of the items, and the rating scale are to be used in their original form. Any modification or unauthorized translation into other languages constitutes a breach of the copyright and violation of basic research ethics (see also User information for the *Acute Recovery and Stress Scale* and the *Short Recovery and Stress Scale*).
3 Inclusion criteria: a maximum strength (estimated one-repetition maximum) of 120% (for male athletes) and 80% (for female athletes) of their own body weight when doing a parallel squat; at least three years of experience in strength training with a frequency of two sessions per week.

6 Comparison of the ARSS and the SRSS

The preceding chapters present the *Acute Recovery and Stress Scale* (ARSS) and *Short Recovery and Stress Scale* (SRSS) as economical and sensitive instruments to measure the current recovery-stress state and their sensitivity to change in the context of sport. They are hence to be seen as separate tools, which can be applied independently or in combination. This chapter highlights the differences between the ARSS and the SRSS and provides a rationale for their use in research and applied settings.

Correlations between the ARSS and the SRSS

Since the SRSS is a derivative of the ARSS that utilizes its items as descriptors, a substantial relationship between these tools should be expected. In the German samples, correlations were moderate to high (GS3, $r_s = .46–.74$; GS5, $r_s = .45–.62$; Table 6.1). The lower correlations for sample GS5, however, support the assumption (as has been stated earlier) that some scales/items were too difficult to understand for the adolescent participants.

Table 6.1 Spearman correlations (r_s) between the equivalent scales/items of the ARSS and the SRSS for samples GS3, GS5, ES1, and ES2

			GS3	GS5			ES1	ES2			
				total	♂	♀		total	ANZ	UK	NA
	Scale/Item	N	574	239	120	119	254	907	375	304	186
Recovery	Physical Performance Capability		.62 a	.62 a	.54 a	.68 a	**.79** a	.69 a	.65 a	.65 a	**.80** a
	Mental Performance Capability		.49 a	.54 a	.45 a	.61 a	.62 a	.68 a	**.71** a	.62 a	.66 a
	Emotional Balance		.46 a	.53 a	.51 a	.55 a	**.71** a	**.75** a	**.73** a	**.75** a	**.79** a
	Overall Recovery		.64 a	.59 a	.55 a	.62 a	.67 a	**.71** a	.68 a	**.73** a	**.72** a
Stress	Muscular Stress		.69 a	.58 a	.50 a	.63 a	.68 a	**.73** a	**.71** a	.65 a	**.83** a
	Lack of Activation		**.74** a	.45 a	.43 a	.48 a	.67 a	**.73** a	**.70** a	**.70** a	**.80** a
	Negative Emotional State		**.70** a	.50 a	.51 a	.47 a	**.75** a	**.77** a	**.80** a	**.74** a	**.79** a
	Overall Stress		.67 a	.56 a	.53 a	.61 a	.64 a	**.73** a	**.72** a	**.70** a	**.78** a

Note: ARSS = *Acute Recovery and Stress Scale*; SRSS = *Short Recovery and Stress Scale*; GS = German sample; ES = English sample; ANZ = Australia/New Zealand; UK = United Kingdom; NA = North America

a = $p < .001$
b = $p < .01$
c = $p < .05$
d = non-significant; $r_s \geq .70$ are bolded

For the English sample ES1, stronger correlations between the ARSS and SRSS scales/items were revealed ($r_s = .62–.79$). Similar values but a reduced range of correlations were observed for ES2 ($r_s = .68–.77$). However, when calculating Spearman correlations separately for the subsamples, Australia/New Zealand showed a range between $r_s = .65$ and $r_s = .80$, the United Kingdom a range between $r_s = .62$ and $r_s = .75$, and the North American a range between $r_s = .66$ and .83.

The morning surveys of sample GS4 showed medium to strong correlations between the items of the SRSS and the scales of the ARSS (Table 6.2). No scale/item showed a consistent correlation, e.g., the correlation for *Mental Performance Capability* varied between $r_s = .49$ and .79. The consistently strongest correlations were found for *Muscular Stress* and *Overall Stress*.

Table 6.2 Spearman correlations (r_s) between the corresponding ARSS scales and SRSS items in sample GS4

	Scale/Item	Day 1 (n = 23)	Day 2 (n = 24)	Day 3 (n = 25)	Day 4 (n = 25)	Day 5 (n = 25)
Recovery	Physical Performance Capability	.64 [a]	.66 [a]	.44 [c]	**.80** [a]	.63 [a]
	Mental Performance Capability	**.74** [a]	**.76** [a]	**.72** [a]	.49 [c]	**.79** [a]
	Emotional Balance	.69 [a]	**.80** [a]	.65 [a]	**.87** [a]	**.70** [a]
	Overall Recovery	**.77** [a]	.66 [a]	.52 [b]	**.83** [a]	**.73** [a]
Stress	Muscular Stress	**.74** [a]	**.73** [a]	**.84** [a]	**.92** [a]	**.79** [a]
	Lack of Activation	.66 [a]	.42 [c]	.66 [a]	**.81** [a]	.65 [a]
	Negative Emotional State	.37 [d]	.57 [b]	**.73** [a]	**.79** [a]	.57 [b]
	Overall Stress	**.89** [a]	**.75** [a]	**.85** [a]	**.90** [a]	**.70** [a]

Note: ARSS = *Acute Recovery and Stress Scale*; SRSS = *Short Recovery and Stress Scale*; r_s = Spearman's rank correlations; Day 1 = Beginning of the training camp and measurement in the evening; otherwise measurements in the morning

[a] = $p < .001$
[b] = $p < .01$
[c] = $p < .05$
[d] = non-significant; $r_s \geq .70$ are bolded; modified from Hitzschke et al. (2016)

In addition to the results displayed in Tables 6.1 and 6.2, in sample GS7, correlations of the German SRSS were calculated intra-individually in seven athletes over a period of 64–65 days, and a similar pattern was observed (Liebscher, 2014). In the *Short Recovery Scale*, these intra-individual correlations were between $r_s = .66$ and .94 for *Physical Performance Capability*, between $r_s = .65$ and .93 for *Mental Performance Capability*, between $r_s = .55$ and .90 for *Emotional Balance*, and the values for *Overall Recovery* were between $r_s = .64$ and .92. Likewise, the correlations within the *Short Stress Scale* were between $r_s = .72$ and .94 for *Muscular Stress*, between $r_s = .63$ and .93 for *Lack of Activation*, between $r_s = .59$ and .90 for *Negative Emotional State*, and between $r_s = .73$ and .92 for *Overall Stress*. Again, the highest correlations were found for *Muscular Stress* and *Overall Stress*.

The English ARSS scales and SRSS items showed similar but not identical correlations with the respective scales/items across different samples. Overall, the English ARSS scales and SRSS items showed higher correlations compared with the original German versions.

Comparison of construct validity

Regarding correlations with the POMS, the RESTQ-Sport-76, and the DOMS, a similar pattern could be revealed for the ARSS and the SRSS. Only one difference ($\Delta \geq .2$) could be observed for the POMS *Anger* and ARSS/SRSS *Overall Stress* (ARSS, $r_s = .40$; SRSS, $r_s = .60$) for sample ES2 (see Tables 4.12 and 5.10).

For sample ES1 (see Tables 4.10 and 5.8), differences in the height of the correlation ($\Delta < .2$) were visible, e.g., between the ARSS scales/SRSS items *Muscular Stress* and the RESTQ-Sport-76 scale *Conflicts/Pressure* (ARSS, $r_s = .19$; SRSS, $r_s = .09$) and *Injury* (ARSS, $r_s = .52$; SRSS, $r_s = .38$), as well as between *General Stress* and *Overall Stress* (ARSS, $r_s = .35$; SRSS, $r_s = .46$). Furthermore, in 11 out of 19 scales of the RESTQ-Sport-76, different heights of correlations ($\Delta < .2$) occurred with *Physical Performance Capability* (in the ARSS/SRSS). For sample ES2 (see Tables 4.10 and 5.8) and the subsamples (see Tables 4.11 and 5.9), only marginal differences in the height of the correlation between the ARSS scales/SRSS items and the RESTQ-Sport-76 scales occurred.

Importantly, similar correlations (Tables 4.12 and 5.10) were found for the scale/item *Muscular Stress* when comparing DOMS with the German ARSS scales/SRSS items (ARSS, $r_s = .59$; SRSS, $r_s = .56$).

Even though the correlations were, in most cases, slightly lower for the SRSS, a similar correlation pattern was observed between the ARSS/SRSS and the RESTQ-Sport-76, as well as for the ARSS/SRSS and DOMS. In both measures (ARSS and SRSS), the highest correlations were found with the scales/items that had similar contents (e.g., *Muscular Stress/Injury*; *Physical Performance Capability/Being in Shape*; *Negative Emotional State/Emotional Stress*). This supports the convergent and construct validity and the content-related conception of both tools.

Comparison of sensitivity to change

Hitzschke et al. (2017) analyzed the intra-individual change and criterion sensitivity of the ARSS and the SRSS in response to a six-day microcycle of intensified strength training (STM) and high-intensity interval training (HIIT) compared with the change in the criterion measures of maximal dynamic strength (estimated 1-repetition maximum [1RMest]; STM) or repeated sprint ability (RSA; HIIT). As a second aim, the results of the subjective measures were compared descriptively with earlier reported physiological and performance markers of the same study (Raeder et al., 2016; Wiewelhove et al., 2015).

The samples consisted of 23 (STM; M = 23.7 ± 2.0 years) and 22 (HIIT; M = 22.8 ± 2.6) well-trained athletes who completed 11 training sessions during the six days to induce a functional overload. The ARSS and the SRSS were completed every morning and the two criterion measures were assessed three times (Pre, $Post_1$, $Post_2$). Effects of training for the whole six-day period and changes from pre- to post-training, as well as after 72 hours of recovery were evaluated (Figure 6.1). In response to the physical stress stimulus in both training protocols, large change effects were found in the overall and physical-related scales/items. Moderate to large change effects were visible in the scales/items that described mental factors, and moderate change effects were shown in the scales/items that described emotional states.

Figure 6.2 shows the daily scores of the ARSS scales separately for HIIT and STM. Among the *Recovery* dimension, the physically oriented scales *Physical Performance Capability* and *Overall Recovery* showed a decline during the microcycle in both training groups, while *Mental Performance Capability* and *Emotional Balance* showed little variation. As day 5 was the only day with one training session instead of two, there was a slight improvement of *Physical Performance Capability* and *Overall Recovery* in the HIIT group from days 5 to 6. Regarding the *Stress* dimension, *Muscular Stress* showed the highest scores among HIIT as well as STM, followed by *Overall Stress* scores. As found in the *Recovery* dimension, a similar small recovery response on day 6 could be interpreted for the HIIT group, due to observed reductions in the *Stress* dimension.

Daily scores of the SRSS showed similar trends to the ARSS scores (Figure 6.3), while more marked variations were visible among *Lack of Activation* and *Negative Emotional State*.

The highest diagnostic effectiveness was also revealed in the overall (45.5–73.9%) and physical-related (45.5–69.9%) scales/items with sensitivity analyses, but they did not differentiate between athletes in a fatigued or recovered state compared to the performance criterion measures. No significant relationships between changes in the scales/items and in the criterion measures were revealed with correlation analyses either. Psychological markers are of high importance for the assessment of recovery and stress. This relevance can be underlined through comparisons with the change effect sizes and the sensitivity results of the performance and physiological markers. By using the ARSS and the SRSS, experiences can be gained regarding the application and evaluation, e.g., the tools are most practical and economical when a combination of subjective and objective markers is used for training monitoring in sport.

Discussion of the ARSS and the SRSS

The ARSS proved to have a better scale homogeneity and item-total correlation compared to the SRSS. However, the results of the SRSS have to be regarded as satisfactory, too. The items of the SRSS and the adjectives of the ARSS are both characterized by an appropriate item mean, dispersion and item-total correlation. The *Short Recovery Scale* and the *Short Stress Scale* of the SRSS and the scales of the ARSS both show a good homogeneity. Intercorrelations exist but are below .85 in both methods, so that a falsification of the results due to collinearity can be excluded. The height of the correlation is also influenced by the calculation of the scores. It needs to be considered that the individual ARSS scores can have .00, .25, .50, or .75 after the full number; on the SRSS, only full numbers can be scored.

By answering 32 single adjectives, more detailed information can be derived from the ARSS than from the SRSS. This had already been implied in the validation studies, particularly by the sensitivity to change of the emotional and mental levels and by the slight advantages in the construct validity with the RESTQ-Sport-76. The SRSS with its more economical design, on the other hand, offers advantages especially when a more frequent measurement is required (e.g., long-term athlete monitoring in training camps; Horvath & Röthlin, 2018). The sensitivity to change and construct validity of the SRSS were within a good range in all items and hardly any differences on the general and physical levels could be detected when compared to the ARSS. Validity could be verified for both questionnaires by conducting field and laboratory studies. Moreover, both methods showed a close reference to theory and fulfilled the request from sports practice of short and economical instruments.

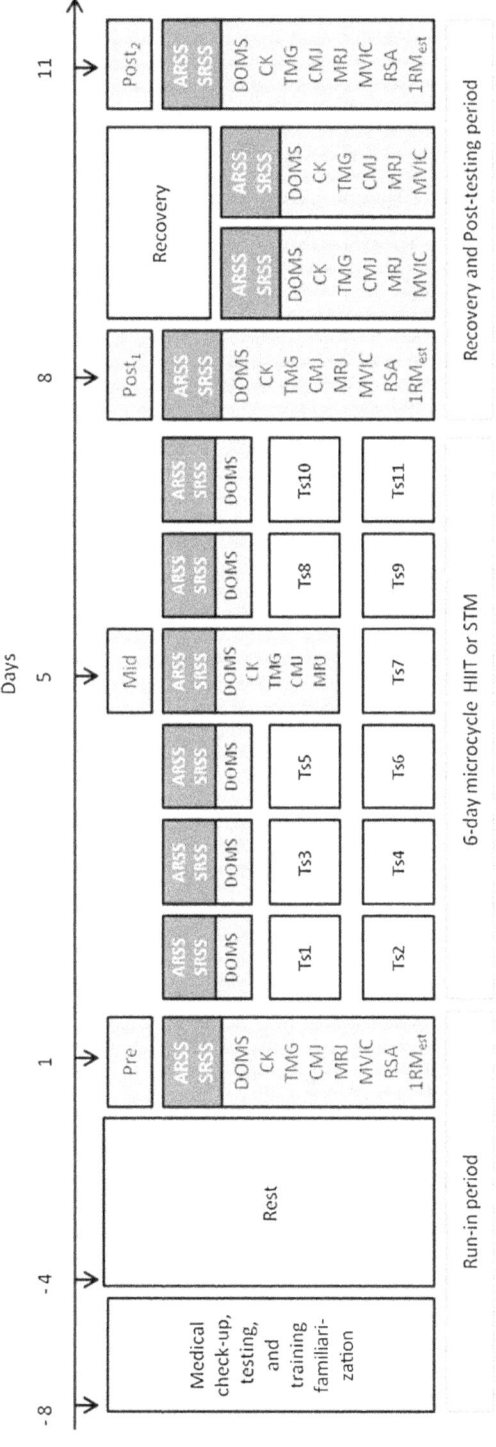

Figure 6.1 Schematic representation of the study design

Note: STM = Strength training microcycle; HIIT = High-intensity interval training; DOMS = Delayed-Onset Muscle Soreness; ARSS = *Acute Recovery and Stress Scale;* SRSS = *Short Recovery and Stress Scale;* CK = Creatine kinase; TMG = Tensiomyography measurements; CMJ = Counter Movement Jump; MRJ = Multiple Rebound Jumps; MVIC = Maximal Voluntary Isometric Contraction; RSA = Repeated Sprint Ability; 1RMest = Estimated 1 Repetition Maximum; Ts = Training session. The dark gray marked methods (ARSS and SRSS) were evaluated by Hitzschke et al. (2017). The light gray-marked methods were evaluated by Wiewelhove et al. (2015) and Raeder et al. (2016).

Source: reprinted, with permission, from Hitzschke et al., 2017, p. 150

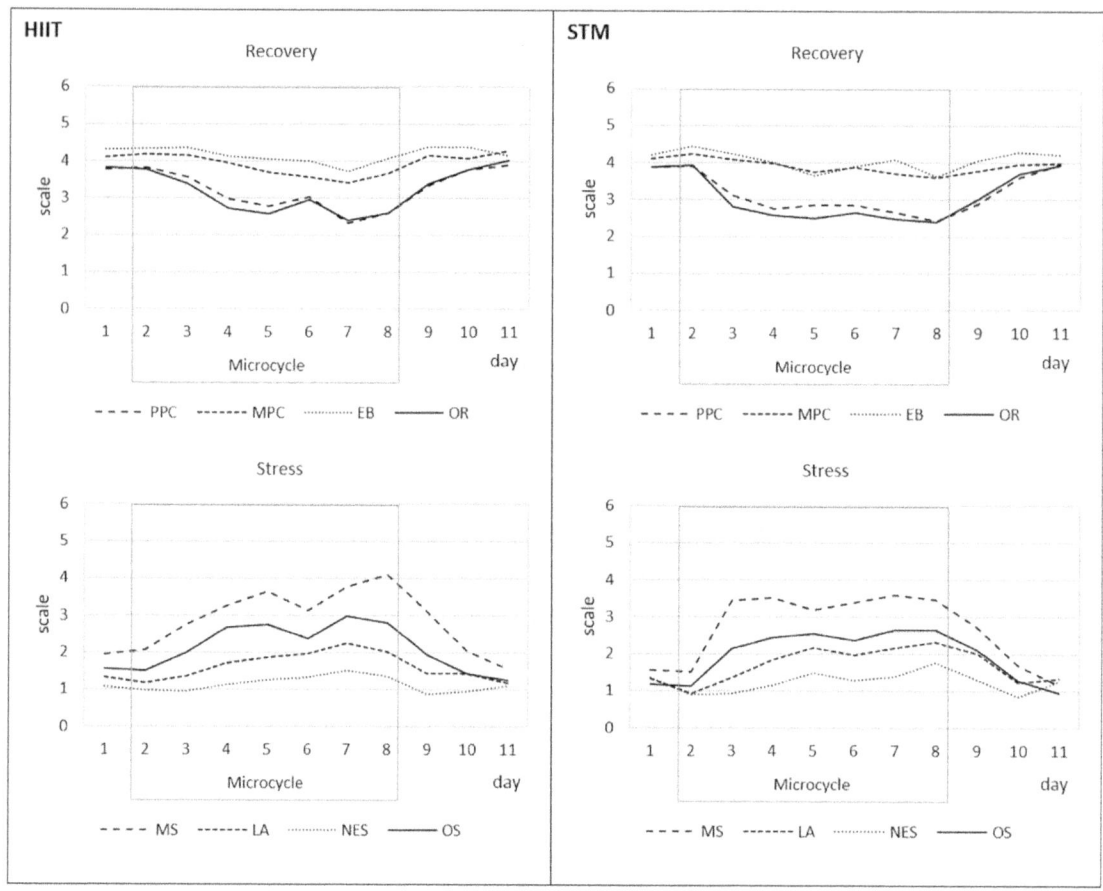

Figure 6.2 Daily scores of the ARSS scales for STM and HIIT

Note: ARSS = *Acute Recovery and Stress Scale*; STM = Strength training microcycle; HIIT = High-intensity interval training; PPC = *Physical Performance Capability*; MPC = *Mental Performance Capability*; EB = *Emotional Balance*; OR = *Overall Recovery*; MS = *Muscular Stress*; LA = *Lack of Activation*; NES = *Negative Emotional State*; OS = *Overall Stress*. The gray frame indicates the days of the training microcycle

Source: reprinted, with permission, from Hitzschke et al., 2017, p. 152

Recommendation for usage in practice

Both the ARSS and SRSS can be used for a long-term athlete monitoring. Due to its compactness, the SRSS can give a quick and easily retraceable feedback about the athlete's current recovery-stress state and changes over time, if baseline measurements are made. It is, however, recommended to let athletes fill in the ARSS before they work with the SRSS. This should be done to familiarize the athlete with the survey mode and the items. If both tools are completed at the same time, an appropriate group size allows correlation coefficients to be calculated between the ARSS and SRSS. This would allow to evaluate the relationship of both tools for a specific sample.

Depending on the objective or research question, the ARSS offers a more detailed picture of the recovery-stress state by answering single adjectives. Within the SRSS item format, the adjectives are only used as descriptors. This is especially the case for the scales that measure emotional states. If a long-term monitoring is intended, it is recommended to use a combination of the ARSS and the SRSS. As is the standard in all psychological methods, it is necessary to inform the athletes about the usage, the advantage, and the significance for an optimum training regulation to prevent 'blurred' values. Moreover, feedback processes should be established as well (Kellmann & Beckmann, 2003; Saw et al., 2017).

Overall, the ARSS and the SRSS can be judged as a valuable addition to the psychometric monitoring of the athlete's recovery-stress state. A combination of the ARSS and the SRSS with the

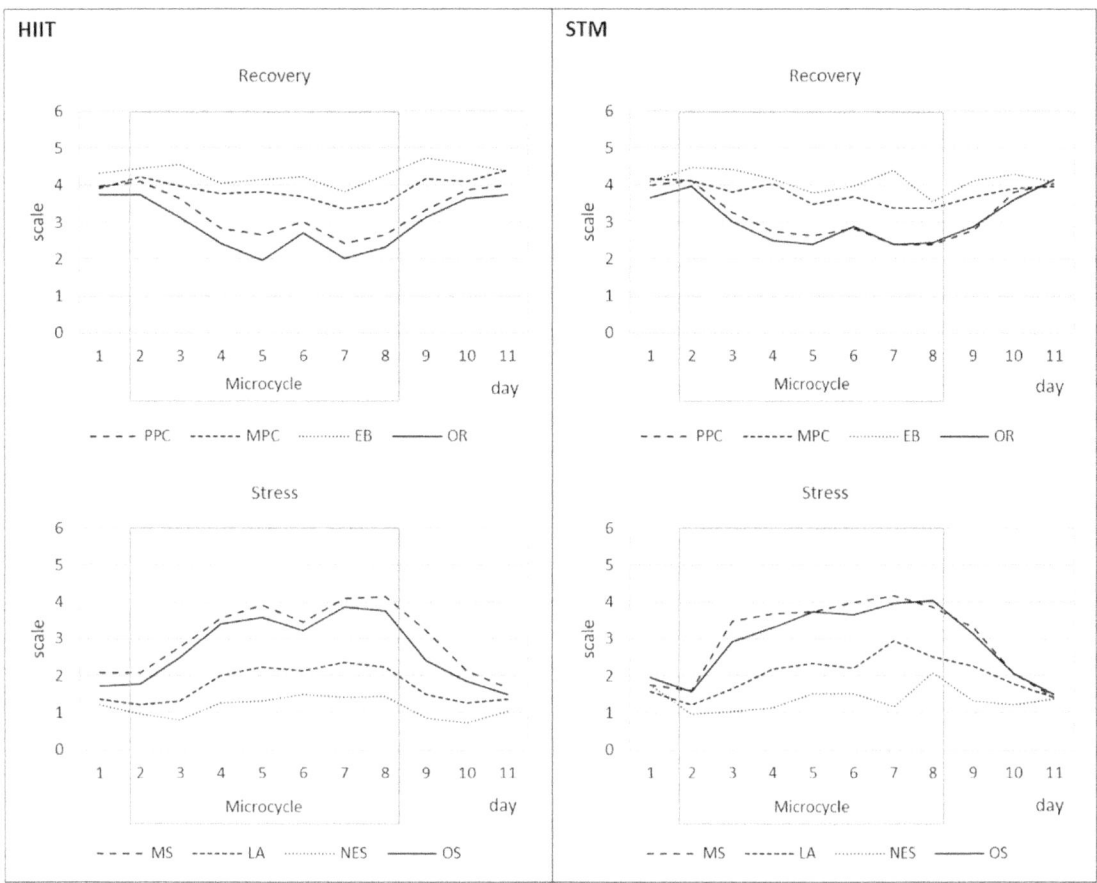

Figure 6.3 Daily scores of the SRSS items for STM and HIIT

Note: SRSS = *Short Recovery and Stress Scale*; STM = Strength training microcycle; HIIT = High-intensity interval training; PPC = *Physical Performance Capability*; MPC = *Mental Performance Capability*; EB = *Emotional Balance*; OR = *Overall Recovery*; MS = *Muscular Stress*; LA = *Lack of Activation*; NES = *Negative Emotional State*; OS = *Overall Stress*. The gray frame indicates the days of the training microcycle

Source: reprinted, with permission, from Hitzschke et al., 2017, p. 154

RESTQ-Sport-76 would complement the acute assessment of state offered by the ARSS and SRSS with aspects that are relevant to behavior/activities regarding the past three days and nights provided by the RESTQ-Sport-76. For a short overview, the characteristics of all three instruments are summarized in Table 6.3.

Table 6.3 Comparison of the ARSS, SRSS, and RESTQ-Sport for the assessment of the recovery-stress state (based on Kellmann et al., 2016)

Area	ARSS	SRSS	RESTQ-Sport
Number of items	32	8	76 / 36
Duration	4–5 min.	40–60 sec.	8–10 min. / 4–5 min.
Economy	++	+++	+/++
Reliability	+++	++	+++
Validity	+++	++	+++
Acute recovery-stress state	+++	+++	+

Table 6.3 (Continued)

Area	ARSS	SRSS	RESTQ-Sport
Measurement in time course			
Frequently daily	++	+++	x
Daily	+++	+++	x
Weekly	+++	+++	+++
Long-term monitoring	+++	+++	+++
Training context			
Training camp	+++	+++	+++
Competition preparation	+++	+++	+++
Training cycles	+++	+++	+
Individual diagnostic	+++	+++	+++
Group diagnostic	+++	+++	+++
Main advantage	economic and simultaneously differentiated, valid assessment	based on its economic use, a high frequent application (frequently daily) is possible	very differentiated recovery-stress balance
Main disadvantage	limited frequent daily use	loss of information through item reduction (i.e., emotional area)	extensive and retrospective assessment (past three days/nights)

Note: ARSS = *Acute Recovery and Stress Scale*; SRSS = *Short Recovery and Stress Scale*; RESTQ-Sport = *Recovery-Stress Questionnaire for Athletes*

+++ = very good applicable
++ = good applicable
+ = applicable with limitations
x = not applicable

Conclusion

The ARSS and the SRSS are useful tools for applied sport psychologists, researchers, physicians, coaches, and athletic trainers. The tools are also valuable for athletes as they allow them to monitor their recovery-stress state and later evaluate how it influences their performance.

- ARSS and SRSS are two theory-based and independent tools.
- ARSS and SRSS fulfill accepted properties of test quality, especially reliability, validity, sensitivity to change, and economy.
- ARSS and SRSS show construct validity with the RESTQ-Sport-76, the POMS, and the DOMS.
- ARSS and SRSS can be used for short-term and long-term athlete monitoring.
- The ARSS is characterized by a detailed assessment of the recovery-stress state; however, the usage per day may be limited, as it consists of 32 items.
- The SRSS can be used for frequently and acutely monitoring athletes; however, the reduction to only eight items leads to a loss of information about the athlete's recovery-stress states.
- It is recommended to use a combination of the ARSS and the SRSS, especially when implementing this type of questionnaire for the first time.

7 Case studies

A balanced recovery-stress state has become more important across the season, due to the big effort (in terms of training and non-football-related activities) young football players are putting into their sport. This became evident during a sport-psychological supervision of a junior Bundesliga team (highest German league for this age group). During this four-week supervision, several 16-year-old players had to fill in the *Short Recovery and Stress Scale* (SRSS) every morning after waking up. The diagnostic investigation of the team offered the following results: Figure 7.1 shows, that during the course of four weeks, the physiological-oriented items for recovery (*Physical Performance Capability*) and stress (*Muscular Stress*), as well as the general items (*Overall Recovery* and *Overall Stress*), reacted to the stress of the match days in the team's mean value (see match day lines in Figure 7.1).

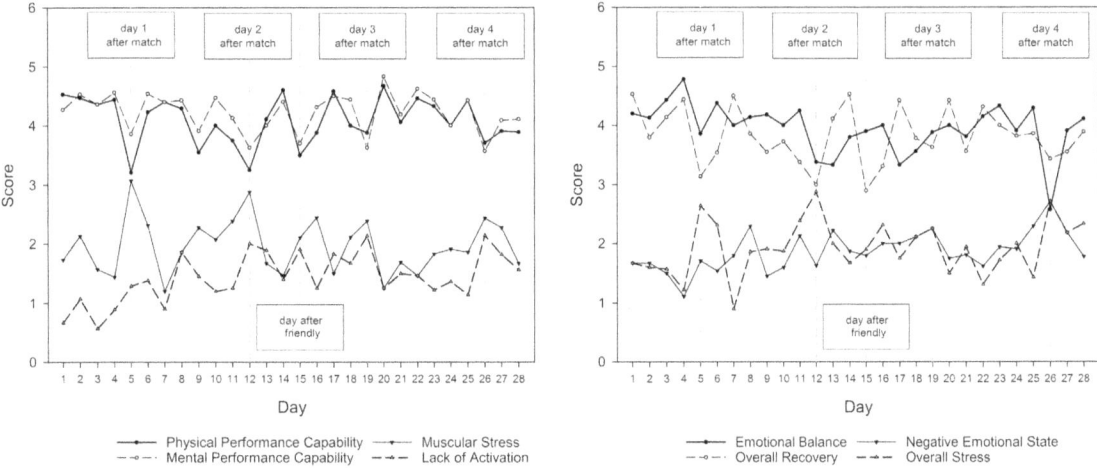

Figure 7.1 Change over time for the *Short Recovery and Stress Scale* items of the football team

Moreover, it shows that two days after match day, stress values decreased and recovery values increased again. It can be concluded that coaches should consider the stress after match days and allow an appropriate regeneration phase. In case of extreme or unexpected values, the analysis of the athletes' values can help coaches to intervene quickly and specifically. The items which focus on the mental state (*Mental Performance Capability* and *Lack of Activation*) and those items which focus on emotional states (*Emotional Balance* and *Negative Emotional State*) vary without a noticeable pattern. An exception, however, is day 26 of the study, as on this day the emotional-oriented items reacted to the match day. In this specific case, after a highly combative and great performance against an opponent with a better placing in the table, the match ended in an unfortunate defeat. In the following training week, the head coach and the sport psychologist focused on the positive aspects of the match, so, despite the defeat, the self-confidence of the players did not decrease, and the team won the next match.

When looking at the players' individual item progression, further conclusions can be drawn. Two situations which were observed during the monitoring will serve as examples. In these two cases, conspicuous values were found in different items of the SRSS.

64 *Case studies*

Case study 1

Within the scope of the described supervision of the youth football team, one player's values in the item *Negative Emotional State* changed drastically and for a longer time from day 13 onwards (Figure 7.2).

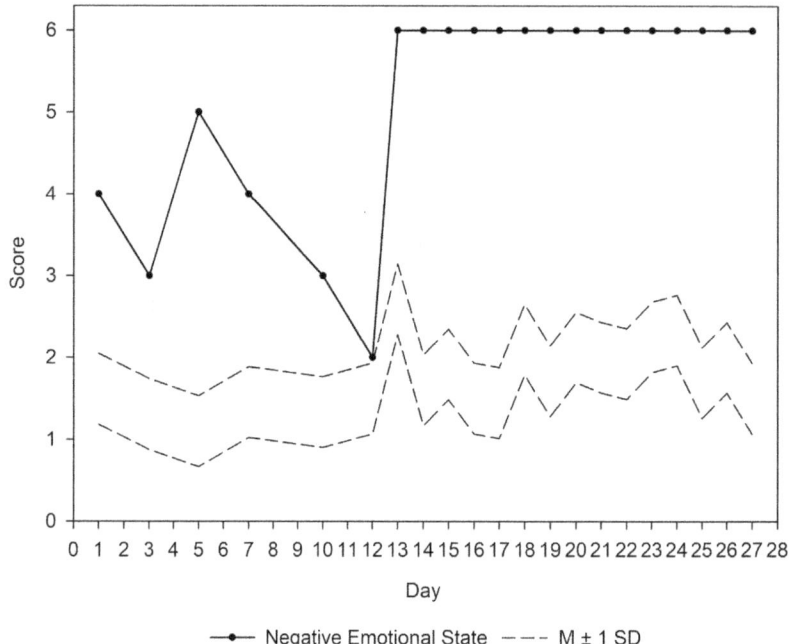

Figure 7.2 Change over time for the *Short Stress Scale* item *Negative Emotional State* and the group mean ± 1 standard deviation for case study 1. Assessment points are represented by the dots

The values were out of the tolerance range for the group as a whole (mean value ± 1 standard deviation) for more than two weeks. Based on this observation, the responsible sport psychologist approached the player. In the following individual consultation, a conflict within the team was recognized and processed. The players were confronted about the situation, asked to give their perspective and, following to the intervention, the conflict was sorted out. After the discrepancies were out of the way, the situation went back to normal for the troubled player and he could successfully play in the last matches of the first half of the season. In this case, the progression chart could be used adequately as a conversation basis for further consultation and intervention.

Case study 2

Case study 2 serves as another example. His progression charts show a steady decrease of the values for the items *Physical Performance Capability* and *Overall Recovery*, until they reach their lowest values on day 27 (Figure 7.3). In the afternoon of this day, the player got injured. After first interviews, it turned out that the player could not cope as well with the additional training sessions in the representative teams and in other youth teams of the club as was initially predicted. It especially became evident that the intensity in the additional two age groups was perceived as much more demanding than expected. In this special case, an adaptation to the stress regulation could potentially have prevented an injury.

Case study 3

Case study 3 is a reserve goalkeeper of a German women's Bundesliga football team who completed the SRSS before and after training (Figure 7.4 [left]) and on the morning before and after a match (Figure 7.4 [right]). While the effects of a training session were recorded as a reduction in *Emotional Balance, Overall*

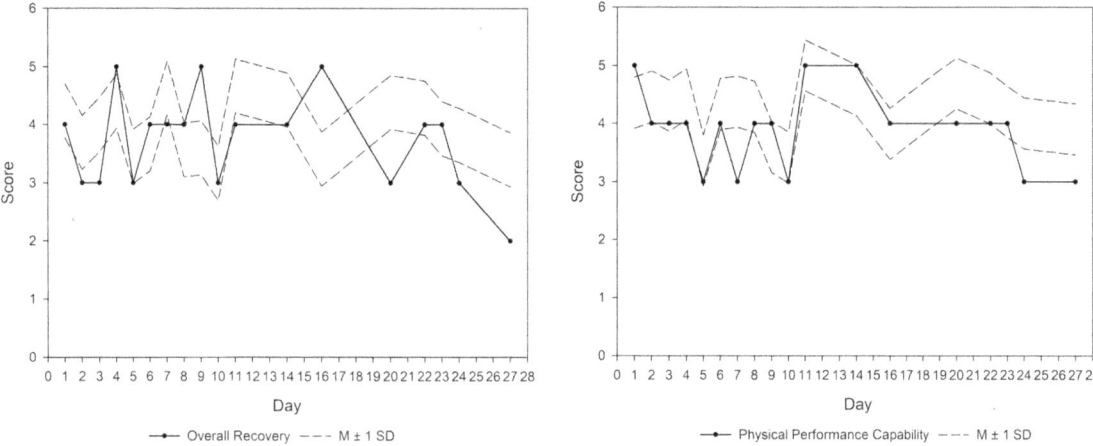

Figure 7.3 Change over time for the *Short Recovery Scale* items *Overall Recovery* [left] and *Physical Performance Capability* [right] and the group mean ± 1 standard deviation for case study 2. Assessment points are represented by the dots

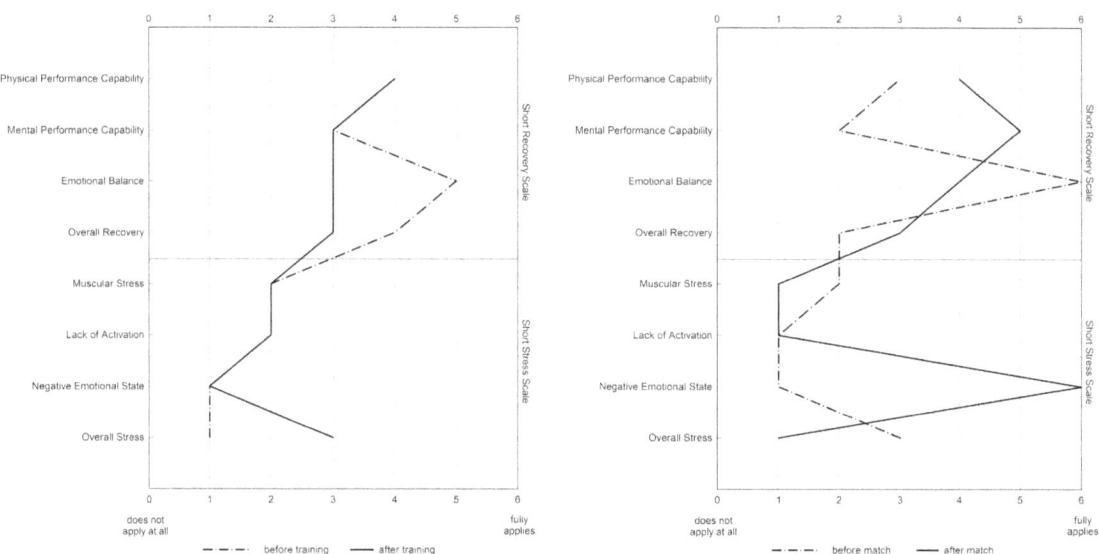

Figure 7.4 Change over time for the *Short Recovery and Stress Scale* items before and after training [left] and the morning before and after a match [right] for case study 3

Recovery and an increase in *Overall Stress*, rather drastic changes could be observed when comparing the scores before and after a Bundesliga match.

It has to be noted that a reserve goalkeeper's chance to play in a match typically only arises if the regular goalkeeper gets injured before or during the match or performs really poorly during the match. In this case, there was a realistic chance for the reserve goalkeeper to play because the regular goalkeeper got injured pre-match and it was uncertain whether she could play in that match. In addition, the team played against a direct opponent to remain in the league and the substitute returned from a long-term injury herself. This obviously affected her emotions quite dramatically, which resulted in high scores in all three items: *Negative Emotional State*, *Physical Performance Capability* and *Mental Performance Capability*. In short, she was ready to perform but also emotionally affected by the uncertainty of her possible chance to play. In the end, she did not play, and after the match some of the scores almost turned to the opposite end of the scale.

66 *Case studies*

Besides these changes in the emotions, *Physical Performance Capability* and *Mental Performance Capability* were also reduced – a good example of how emotional components with a potential worry element can affect the personal assessment of physical and mental performance capability. From an intervention perspective, the pre-match assessment could call on the coach or sport psychologist to intervene in order to increase self-efficacy and remind and refresh the player's performance capabilities.

Case study 4

For the monitoring of acute recovery and stress states in a professional Australian Rules football team throughout the season, the ARSS was used to identify players who should receive additional attention. With the help of a longitudinal representation of data, group means and changes were made noticeable and players who differed from group means were identified easily. Figure 7.5 visualizes lower *Mental Performance Capability* for one case study compared with the group mean and standard deviation throughout most of the season.

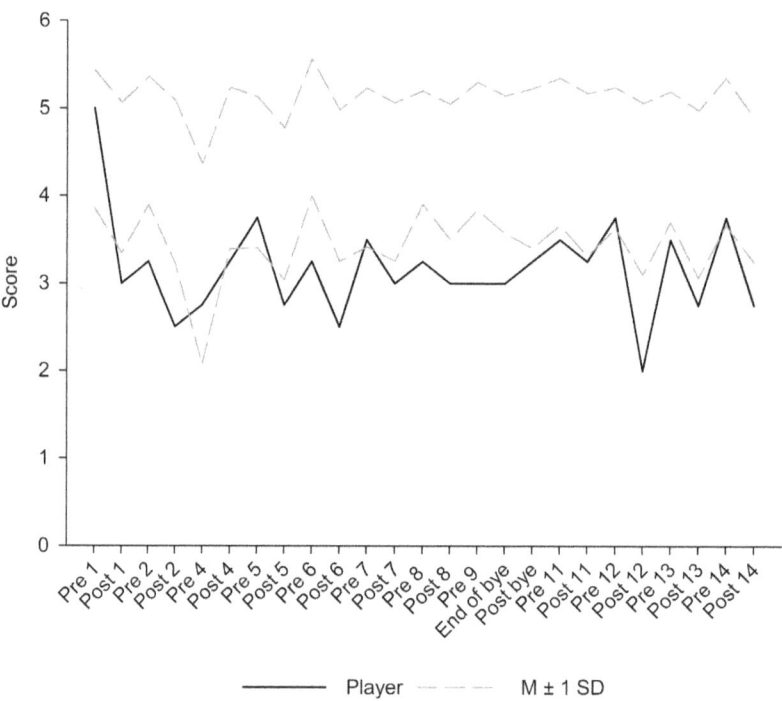

Figure 7.5 Case example of *Mental Performance Capability* for one individual player throughout the matches of the season. Dashed lines represent group mean average ± one standard deviation. The solid line exemplifies values for case study 4

Note: Pre = Pre-match; Post = Post-match; Bye describes a week without a game

Given the consistently lower *Mental Performance Capability* during the week, both after (48 hours) and before (24 hours) competition (capturing the start and end of the training week), ARSS monitoring is an easily applicable approach and starting point for further investigation of causes for a decline in *Mental Performance Capability* and resulting interventions.

References

Anderson, J. C., & Gerbing, D. W. (1988). Structural equation modeling in practice: A review and recommended two-step approach. *Psychological Bulletin, 103*(3), 411–423.

Auersperger, I., Škof, B., Leskošek, B., Knap, B., Jerin, A., Lainščak, M., & Kajtna, T. (2014). Biochemical, hormonal and psychological monitoring of eight weeks endurance running training program in female runners. *Kinesiology: International Journal of Fundamental and Applied Kinesiology, 46*(S1), S30–S39.

Beauducel, A., & Wittmann, W. W. (2005). Simulation study on fit indexes in CFA based on data with slightly distorted simple structure. *Structural Equation Modeling, 12*(1), 41–75.

Borg, G. (1998). *Borg's Perceived Exertion and Pain Scale*. Champaign, IL: Human Kinetics.

Bouget, M., Rouveix, M., Michaux, O., Pequignot, J.-M., & Filaire, E. (2006). Relationships among training stress, mood and dehydroepiandrosterone sulphate/cortisol ratio in female cyclists. *Journal of Sports Sciences, 24*, 1297–1302.

Bresciani, G., Cuevas, M. J., Molinero, O., Almar, M., Suay, F., Salvador, A., de Paz, J. A., Marquez, S., & Gonzáles-Gallego, J. (2011). Signs of overload after an intensified training. *International Journal of Sports Medicine, 32*, 338–343.

Brink, M. S., Visscher, C., Coutts, A. J., & Lemmink, K. A. (2012). Changes in perceived stress and recovery in over-reached young elite soccer players. *Scandinavian Journal of Medicine & Science in Sports, 22*, 285–292.

Brown, H., Dawson, B., Binnie, M. J., Pinnington, H., Sim, M., Clemons, T. D., & Peeling, P. (2017). Sand training: Exercise-induced muscle damage and inflammatory responses to matched-intensity exercise. *European Journal of Sport Science, 17*, 741–747.

Browne, M., & Cudeck, R. (1993). Alternative ways of assessing equation. In K. Bollen & J. Long (Eds.), *Testing structural equation models* (pp. 136–162). Newbury Park, CA: Sage.

Bühner, M. (2011). *Einführung in die Test- und Fragebogenkonstruktion* [Introduction into test- and questionnaire construction]. München: Pearson Studium.

Byrne, B. M. (2001). *Structural equation modeling with AMOS: Basic concepts, applications, and programming*. Mahwah, NJ: Erlbaum.

Cleather, D. J., & Guthrie, S. R. (2007). Quantifying delayed-onset muscle soreness: A comparison of unidimensional and multidimensional instrumentation. *Journal of Sports Sciences, 25*, 845–850.

Collette, R. (2016). *Trainings- und Erholungsmonitoring im Leistungssport Schwimmen* [Training and recovery monitoring in high-performance swimming]. Hamburg: Kovac.

Collette, R., Kellmann, M., Ferrauti, A., Meyer, T., & Pfeiffer, M. (2018). Relation between training load and recovery-stress state in high-performance swimming. *Frontiers in Physiology, 9*, 845. DOI: 10.3389/fphys.2018.00845

Coutts, A. J., Crowcroft, S., & Kempton, T. (2018). Developing athlete monitoring systems: Theoretical basis and practical applications. In M. Kellmann & J. Beckmann (Eds.), *Sport, recovery, and performance: Interdisciplinary insights* (pp. 19–32). Abingdon: Routledge.

Coutts, A. J., Wallace, L. K., & Slattery, K. M. (2007). Monitoring changes in performance, physiology, biochemistry and psychology during overreaching and recovery in triathletes. *International Journal of Sports Medicine, 28*, 125–134.

Diener, E., & Emmons, R. (1984). The interdependence of positive and negative affect. *Journal of Personality and Social Psychology, 47*, 105–117.

di Fronso, S., Nakamura, F. Y., Bortoli, L., Robazza, C., & Bertollo, M. (2013). Stress and recovery balance in amateur basketball players: Differences by gender and preparation phase. *International Journal of Sports Physiology and Performance, 8*, 618–622.

dos Santos, P. B., Kuczynski, K. M., Machado, T. A., Osiecki, A. C. V., & Stefanello, J. M. F. (2014). Psychophysiological stress in under-17 soccer players. *Journal of Exercise Physiologoy Online, 17*(2), 67–80.

Dupont, G., Nédélec, M., McCall, A., McCormack, D., Berthoin, S., & Wisloff, U. (2010). Effect of 2 soccer matches in a week on physical performance and injury rate. *American Journal of Sports Medicine, 38*, 1752–1758.

Ekstrand, J., Walden, M., & Hagglund, M. (2004). A congested football calendar and the wellbeing of players: Correlation between match exposure of European footballers before the World Cup 2002 and their injuries and performances during that World Cup. *British Journal of Sports Medicine, 38*, 493–497.

Foster, C. (1998). Monitoring training in athletes with reference to overtraining syndrome. *Medicine and Science in Sports and Exercise, 30*, 1164–1168.

Fürntratt, E. (1969). Zur Bestimmung der Anzahl interpretierbarer gemeinsamer Faktoren psychologischer Daten [Determining the number of interpretable common factors in factor analyses of psychological data]. *Diagnostica, 15*, 62–75.

Garatachea, N., García-López, D., José Cuevas, M., Almar, M., Molinero, O., Márquez, S., & Gonzáles-Gallego, J. (2011). Biological and psychological monitoring of training status during an entire season in top kayakas. *Journal of Sports Medicine and Physical Fitness, 51*, 339–346.

Halson, S. L. (2014). Monitoring training load to understand fatigue in athletes. *Sports Medicine, 44*(Suppl. 2), 139–147.

Hammes, D., Skorski, S., Schwindling, S., Ferrauti, A., Pfeiffer, M., Kellmann, M., & Meyer, T. (2016). Can the Lamberts and Lambert submaximal cycle test (LSCT) indicate fatigue and recovery in trained cyclists? *International Journal of Sports Physiology and Performance, 11*, 328–336.

Hausswirth, C., & Mujika, I. (Eds.). (2013). *Recovery for performance in sport*. Champaign, IL: Human Kinetics.

Hecksteden, A., Pitsch, W., Julian, R. A., Pfeiffer, M., Kellmann, M., Ferrauti, A., & Meyer, T. (2017). A new method to individualize monitoring of muscle recovery in athletes. *International Journal of Sports Physiology and Performance, 12*, 1137–1142.

Heidari, J., Beckmann, J., Bertollo, M., Brink, M., Kallus, K. W., Robazza, C., & Kellmann, M. (2019). Multidimensional monitoring of recovery and implications for performance. *International Journal of Sports Physiology and Performance, 14*, 2–8.

Heidari, J., Kölling, S., Pelka, M., & Kellmann, M. (2018). Monitoring the recovery-stress state in athletes. In M. Kellmann & J. Beckmann (Eds.), *Sport, recovery, and performance: Interdisciplinary insights* (pp. 3–18). Abingdon: Routledge.

Hitzschke, B., Holst, T., Ferrauti, A., Meyer, T., Pfeiffer, M., & Kellmann, M. (2016). Entwicklung des Akutmaßes zur Erfassung von Erholung und Beanspruchung im Sport [Development of the Acute Recovery and Stress Scale]. *Diagnostica, 62*, 212–226.

Hitzschke, B., Kölling, S., Ferrauti, A., Meyer, T., Pfeiffer, M., & Kellmann, M. (2015). Entwicklung der Kurzskala zur Erfassung von Erholung und Beanspruchung im Sport (KEB) [Development of the Short Recovery and Stress Scale for Sports (SRSS)]. *Zeitschrift für Sportpsychologie, 22*, 146–161.

Hitzschke, B., Wiewelhove, T., Raeder, C., Ferrauti, A., Meyer, T., Pfeiffer, M., Kellmann, M., & Kölling, S. (2017). Evaluation of psychological measures for the assessment of recovery and stress during a shock-microcycle in strength and high-intensity interval training. *Performance Enhancement & Health, 5*, 147–157.

Hoffman, J. R., Epstein, S., Yarom, Y., Zigel, L., & Einbinder, M. (1999). Hormonal and biochemical changes in elite basketball players during a 4-week training camp. *Journal of Strength Condition Research, 13*, 280–285.

Hoffmann, R. M., Müller, T., Hajak, G., & Cassel, W. (1997). Abend-Morgenprotokolle in Schlafforschung und Schlafmedizin – Ein Standardinstrument für den deutschsprachigen Raum [Sleep logs in sleep research and sleep medicine]. *Somnologie, 1*, 103–109.

Homburg, C., & Giering, A. (1996). Konzeptionalisierung und Operationalisierung komplexer Konstrukte – Ein Leitfaden für die Marketingforschung [Conzeptualisation and operalisation of complex constructs: A guidance for marketing research]. *Marketing: Zeitschrift für Forschung und Praxis, 18*(1), 5–24.

Hooper, S. L., Mackinnon, L. T., Howard, A., & Gordon, R. D. (1995). Markers for monitoring overtraining and recovery. *Medicine and Science in Sports and Exercise, 27*, 106–112.

Hortobagyi, T., & Denahan, T. (1989). Variability in creatine kinase: Methodological, exercise and clinically related factors. *International Journal of Sports Medicine, 10*, 69–80.

Horvath, S., & Röthlin, P. (2018). How to improve athletes' return of investment: Shortening questionnaires in the applied sport psychology setting. *Journal of Applied Sport Psychology, 30*, 241–248.

Hough, J., Corney, R., Kouris, A., & Gleeson, M. (2013). Salivary cortisol and testosterone responses to high-intensity cycling before and after an 11-day intensified training period. *Journal of Sports Sciences, 31*, 1614–1623.

Hu, L., & Bentler, P. M. (1999). Cutoff criteria for fit indexes in covariance structure analysis: Conventional criteria versus new alternatives. *Structural Equation Modeling, 6*(1), 1–55.

Impellizzeri, F. M., Rampinini, E., Coutts, A. J., Sassi, A., & Marcora, S. M. (2004). Use of RPE-based training load in soccer. *Medicine and Science in Sports and Exercise, 36*, 1042–1047.

Jagodzinski, W., Kühnel, S. M., & Schmidt, P. (1987). Is there a 'Socratic effect' in nonexperimental panel studies? *Sociological Methods & Research, 15*, 259–302.

Jerusalem, M. (1990). *Persönliche Ressourcen, Vulnerabilität und Streßerleben* [Personal resources, vulnerability, and stress experience]. Göttingen: Hogrefe.

Julian, R. A., Meyer, T., Fullagar, H. H. K., Skorski, S., Kellmann, M., Pfeiffer, M., Ferrauti, A., & Hecksteden, A. (2017). Individual patterns in blood-borne indicators of fatigue-trait or chance. *Journal of Strength and Conditioning Research, 31*, 608–619.

Kallus, K. W. (2016). Stress and recovery: An overview. In K. W. Kallus & M. Kellmann (Eds.), *The Recovery-Stress Questionnaires: User manual* (pp. 27–48). Frankfurt am Main: Pearson Assessment & Information GmbH.

Kellmann, M. (2002). Psychological assessment of underrecovery. In M. Kellmann (Ed.), *Enhancing recovery: Preventing underperformance in athletes* (pp. 37–55). Champaign, IL: Human Kinetics.

Kellmann, M. (2010). Preventing overtraining in athletes in high-intensity sports and stress/recovery monitoring. *Scandinavian Journal of Medicine & Science in Sports, 20*, 95–102.

Kellmann, M., Altenburg, D., Lormes, W., & Steinacker, J. M. (2001). Assessing stress and recovery during preparation for the World Championships in rowing. *The Sport Psychologist, 15*, 151–167.

Kellmann, M., & Beckmann, J. (2003). Research and intervention in sport psychology: New perspectives on an inherent conflict. *International Journal of Sport and Exercise Psychology, 1*, 13–26.

Kellmann, M., & Beckmann, J. (Eds.). (2018a). *Sport, recovery, and performance: Interdisciplinary insights*. Abingdon: Routledge.

Kellmann, M., & Beckmann, J. (2018b). Sport, recovery, and performance: A concluding summary. In M. Kellmann & J. Beckmann (Eds.), *Sport, recovery, and performance: Interdisciplinary insights* (pp. 260–265). Abingdon: Routledge.

Kellmann, M., Bertollo, M., Bosquet, L., Brink, M., Coutts, A. J., Duffield, R., Erlacher, D., Halson, S. L., Hecksteden, A., Heidari, J., Kallus, K. W., Meeusen, R., Mujika, I., Robazza, C., Skorski, S., Venter, R., & Beckmann, J. (2018). Recovery and performance in sport: Consensus statement. *International Journal of Sports Physiology and Performance, 13*, 240–245.

Kellmann, M., & Günther, K.-D. (2000). Changes in stress and recovery in elite rowers during preparations for the Olympic Games. *Medicine and Science in Sports and Exercise, 32*, 676–683.

Kellmann, M., & Kallus, K. W. (2001). *Recovery-Stress Questionnaire for Athletes*. Champaign, IL: Human Kinetics.

Kellmann, M., & Kallus, K. W. (2016). The Recovery-Stress Questionnaire for Athletes. In K. W. Kallus & M. Kellmann (Eds.), *The Recovery-Stress Questionnaires: User manual* (pp. 86–131). Frankfurt am Main: Pearson Assessment & Information GmbH.

Kellmann, M., Kölling, S., & Hitzschke, B. (2016). *Das Akutmaß und die Kurzskala zur Erfassung von Erholung und Beanspruchung im Sport –Manual* [The Acute Measure and the Short Scale of Recovery and Stress for Sports: Manual]. Hellenthal: Sportverlag Strauß.

Kellmann, M., Pelka, M., & Beckmann, J. (2018). Psychological relaxation techniques to enhance recovery in sports. In M. Kellmann & J. Beckmann (Eds.), *Sport, recovery, and performance: Interdisciplinary insights* (pp. 247–259). Abingdon: Routledge.

Kenttä, G., & Hassmén, P. (1998). Overtraining and recovery: A conceptual model. *Sports Medicine, 26*, 1–16.

Kölling, S., Hitzschke, B., Holst, T., Ferrauti, A., Meyer, T., Pfeiffer, M., & Kellmann, M. (2015). Validity of the Acute Recovery and Stress Scale: Training monitoring of the German junior national field hockey team. *International Journal of Sports Science & Coaching, 10*, 529–542.

Kölling, S., Steinacker, J. M., Pfeiffer, M., Ferrauti, A., Meyer, T., & Kellmann, M. (2016). The longer the better: Sleep/wake patterns during preparation of the World Rowing Junior Championships. *Chronobiology International, 33*(1), 73–84.

Lamberts, R. P., Swart, J., Noakes, T. D., & Lambert, M. I. (2011). A novel submaximal cycle test to monitor fatigue and predict cycling performance. *British Journal of Sports Medicine, 45*, 797–804.

Laux, P., Krumm, B., Diers, M., & Flor, H. (2015). Recovery-stress balance and injury risk in professional football players: A prospective study. *Journal of Sports Sciences, 33*, 2140–2148.

Lazarus, R. S. (1991). *Emotion and adaptation*. New York, NY: Oxford University Press.

Liebscher, R. (2014). *Das Akutmaß Erholung und Beanspruchung. Ein Vergleich der Kurz- und der Langversion im Hinblick auf die Aussagekraft zur Erfassung der multidimensionalen Aspekte von Erholung und Beanspruchung* [The Acute Recovery and Stress Scale: A comparison of the long and short version for the assessment of multi-dimensional aspects of recovery and stress]. Unpublished Bachelor's Thesis, Johannes Gutenberg-Universität, Mainz.

Lienert, G. A., & Raatz, U. (1998). *Testaufbau und Testanalyse* [Development and analysis of tests]. Weinheim: Beltz, PVU.

Lord, F. M., & Novick, M. R. (1968). *Statistical theories of mental test scores*. Reading, MA: Addison-Wesley.

Mäetsu, J., Jürimäe, J., & Jürimäe, T. (2005). Monitoring of performance and training in rowing. *Sports Medicine, 35*, 597–617.

Main, L., & Landers, G. (2012). Overtertraining or burnout: A training and psycho-behavioural case study. *International Journal of Sports Science and Coaching, 7*(1), 127–128.

Mayring, P. (2010). *Qualitative Inhaltsanalyse* [Qualitative content analysis]. Weinheim: Beltz.

McDonald, R. P., & Ho, M. H. R. (2002). Principal and practice in reporting structural equation analyses. *Psychological Methods, 7*(1), 64–82.

McNair, D. M., Lorr, M., & Droppleman, L. F. (1992). *Revised Manual for the Profile of Mood States*. San Diego, CA: Educational and Industrial Testing Service.

Meeusen, R., & De Pauw, K. (2018). Overtraining: What do we know? In M. Kellmann & J. Beckmann (Eds.), *Sport, recovery, and performance: Interdisciplinary insights* (pp. 51–62). Abingdon: Routledge.

Meeusen, R., Duclos, M., Foster, C., Fry, A., Glesson, M., Nieman, D., Raglin, J., Rietjens, G., Steinacker, J., & Urhausen, A. (2013). Prevention, diagnosis and treatment of the overtraining syndrome: Joint consensus statement of the European College of Sport Science (ECSS) and the American College of Sports Medicine (ACSM). *Medicine and Science in Sports and Exercise, 45*, 186–205.

Meister, S., Faude, O., Amman, T., Schnittker, R., & Meyer, T. (2013). Indicators for high physical strain and overload in elite football players. *Scandinavian Journal of Medicine & Science in Sports, 23*, 156–163.

Meyer, T. (2010). Regeneration im Leistungssport [Regeneration in elite sports]. *Deutsche Zeitschrift für Sportmedizin, 61,* 127–128.

Meyer, T., Ferrauti, A., Kellmann, M., & Pfeiffer, M. (2016). *Regenerationsmanagement im Spitzensport* [Management of regeneration in elite sports]. Köln: Sportverlag Strauß.

Moosbrugger, H. (1982). Dimensionalitätsuntersuchungen von FPI-Skalen mit dem Klassischen Latent-Additiven Testmodell (KLA-Modell) [Dimensionality studies of FPI-scales with the classical latent-additive test model (CLA-model)]. *Zeitschrift für Differentielle und Diagnostische Psychologie, 3,* 241–264.

Nässi, A., Ferrauti, A., Meyer, T., Pfeiffer, M., & Kellmann, M. (2017a). Development of two short measures for recovery and stress in sport. *European Journal of Sport Science, 17,* 894–903.

Nässi, A., Ferrauti, A., Meyer, T., Pfeiffer, M., & Kellmann, M. (2017b). Psychological tools used for monitoring training responses of athletes. *Performance Enhancement & Health, 5,* 125–133.

Nédélec, M., McCall, A., Carling, C., Legall, F., Berthoin, S., & Dupont, G. (2012). Recovery in soccer: Part I: Post-match fatigue and time course of recovery. *Sports Medicine, 42,* 997–1015.

Noble, B., & Robertson, R. J. (1996). *Perceived exertion.* Champaign, IL: Human Kinetics.

Nosaka, K., Newton, M., & Sacco, P. (2002). Delayed-onset muscle soreness does not reflect the magnitude of eccentric exercise-induced muscle damage. *Scandinavian Journal of Medicine & Science in Sports, 12,* 337–346.

O'Connor, B. P. (2000). SPSS and SAS programs for determining the number of components using parallel analysis and Velicer's MAP test. *Behavior Research Methods, Instruments & Computers, 32,* 396–402.

Ohnhaus, E. E., & Adler, R. (1975). Methodological problems in the measurement of pain: A comparison between the verbal rating scale and the visual analogue scale. *Pain, 1,* 379–384.

O'Toole, M. L. (1998). Overreaching and overtraining in endurance athletes. In R. B. Kreider, A. C. Fry, & M. L. O'Toole (Eds.), *Overtraining in sport* (pp. 3–17). Champaign, IL: Human Kinetics.

Otter, R. T. A., Brink, M. S., van der Does, H. T. D., & Lemmink, K. A. (2016). Monitoring perceived stress and recovery in relation to cycling performance in female athletes. *International Journal of Sports Medicine, 37,* 12–18.

Page, W., Swan, R., & Patterson, S. D. (2017). The effect of intermittent lower limb occlusion on recovery following exercise-induced muscle damage: A randomized controlled trial. *Journal of Science and Medicine in Sport, 20,* 729–733.

Pelka, M., Ferrauti, A., Meyer, T., Pfeiffer, M., & Kellmann, M. (2017). How does a short, interrupted recovery break affect performance and how is it assessed? A study on acute effects. *International Journal of Sports Physiology and Performance, 12*(Suppl. 2), S2-114–S2-121.

Pelka, M., & Kellmann, M. (2017). Recovery and relaxation in sport and performance. In O. Braddick (Ed.), *Oxford research encyclopedia of psychology* (pp. 1–22). New York, NY: Oxford University Press.

Pelka, M., Kölling, S., Ferrauti, A., Meyer, T., Pfeiffer, M., & Kellmann, M. (2017). Psychological relaxation between two physical tasks. *Journal of Sports Sciences, 35,* 216–223.

Pelka, M., Schneider, P., & Kellmann, M. (2018). Development of pre- and post-match morning recovery-stress states during in-season weeks in elite youth football. *Science and Medicine in Football, 2,* 127–132.

Puta, C., Steidten, T., Baumbach, P., Wöhrl, T., May, R., Kellmann, M., Herbsleb, M., Gabriel, B., Weber, S., Granacher, U., & Gabriel, H. (2018). Standardized assessment of resistance training-induced subjective symptoms and objective signs of immunological stress responses in young athletes. *Frontiers in Physiology, 9,* 698. DOI: 10.3389/fphys.2018.00698

Raeder, C., Wiewelhove, T., de Paula Simola, R. A., Kellmann, M., Meyer, T., Pfeiffer, M., & Ferrauti, A. (2016). Assessment of fatigue and recovery in male and female athletes following six days of intensified strength training. *Journal of Strength and Conditioning Research, 30,* 3412–3427.

Raglin, J. S. (1993). Overtraining and staleness: Psychometric monitoring of endurance athletes. In R. B. Singer, M. Murphey, & L. K. Tennant (Eds.), *Handbook of research on sport psychology* (pp. 840–850). New York, NY: Macmillan.

Raglin, J. S., Morgan, W. P., & O'Connor, P. J. (1991). Changes in mood states during training in female and male college swimmers. *International Journal of Sports Medicine, 12,* 585–589.

Raglin, J. S., & Wilson, G. S. (2000). Overtraining in athletes. In Y. L. Hanin (Ed.), *Emotions in sport* (pp. 191–207). Champaign, IL: Human Kinetics.

Rohmert, W., & Rutenfranz, J. (1975). *Arbeitswissenschaftliche Beurteilung der Belastung und Beanspruchung an unterschiedlichen industriellen Arbeitsplätzen* [Scientific rating on stress in different industrial work places]. Bonn: Bundesminister für Arbeit und Sozialordnung.

Saw, A. E., Kellmann, M., Main, L. C., & Gastin, P. B. (2017). Athlete self-report measures in research and practice: Recommendations for the discerning reader and fastidious practitioner. *International Journal of Sports Physiology and Performance, 12*(Suppl. 2), S2-127–S2-135.

Saw, A. E., Main, L. C., & Gastin, P. B. (2016). Monitoring the athlete training response: Subjective self-reported measures trump commonly used objective measures: A systematic review. *British Journal of Sports Medicine, 50,* 281–291.

Scherr, J., Wolfarth, B., Christle, J. W., Pressler, A., Wagenpfeil, S., & Halle, M. (2013). Associations between Borg's Rating of Perceived Exertion and physiological measures of exercise intensity. *European Journal of Applied Physiology, 113,* 147–155.

Schimpchen, J., Wagner, M., Ferrauti, A., Kellmann, M., Pfeiffer, M., & Meyer, T. (2017). Can cold water immersion enhance recovery in elite Olympic weightlifters?: An individualized perspective. *Journal of Strength and Conditioning Research, 31*, 1569–1576.

Skovgaard, C., Christensen, P. M., Larsen, S., Rostgaard Andersen, T., Thomassen, M., & Bangsbo, J. (2014). Concurrent speed endurance and resistance training improves performance, running economy, and muscle NHE1 in moderately trained runners. *Journal of Applied Physiology, 117*, 1097–1109.

Slivka, D. R., Hailes, W. S., Cuddy, J. S., & Ruby, B. C. (2010). Effects of 21 days of intensified training on markers of overtraining. *Journal of Strength and Conditioning Research, 24*, 2604–2612.

Snyder, A. C. (1998). Overtraining and glycogen depletion hypothesis. *Medicine and Science in Sports and Exercise, 7*, 1146–1150.

Snyder, A. C., Jeukendrup, A. E., Hesselink, M. K. C., Kuipers, H., & Foster, C. (1993). A physiological/psychological indicator of overreaching during intensive training. *International Journal of Sports Medicine, 14*, 29–32.

Steinacker, J. M., Lormes, W., Lehmann, M., & Altenburg, D. (1998). Training of rowers before World Championships. *Medicine and Science in Sport and Exercise, 30*, 1158–1163.

Ten Haaf, T., van Staveren, S., Oudenhoven, E., Piacentini, M. F., Meeusen, R., Roelands, B., Koenderman, L., Daanen, H. A. M., Foster, C., & de Koning, J. J. (2017). Prediction of functional overreaching from subjective fatigue and readiness to train after only 3 days of cycling. *International Journal of Sports Physiology and Performance, 12*(Suppl. 2), S2-287–S2-294.

Trudgill, P., & Hannah, J. (2017). *International English: A guide to varieties of English around the world*. Abingdon: Routledge.

Urhausen, A., & Kindermann, W. (2002). Diagnosis of overtraining: What tools do we have? *Sports Medicine, 32*, 95–102.

Vallerand, R. J. (1989). Vers une méthodologie de validation transculturelle de questionnaires psychologiques: Implications pour la recherche en langue française [Toward a methodology for the transcultural validation of psychological questionnaires: Implications for research in the French language]. *Canadian Psychology, 30*, 662–680.

van der Does, H. T., Brink, M. S., Otter, R. T., Visscher, C., & Lemmink, K. A. (2017). Injury risk is increased by changes in perceived recovery of team sport players. *Clinical Journal of Sport Medicine, 27*(1), 46–51.

Weiber, R., & Mühlhaus, D. (2010). *Strukturgleichungsmodellierung* [Structural equation modeling]. Heidelberg: Springer.

West, S. G., Finch, J. F., & Curran, P. J. (1995). Structural equation models with nonnormal variables: Problems and remedies. In R. Hoyle (Ed.), *Structural equation modeling: Concepts, issues, and applications* (pp. 56–75). Thousand Oaks, CA: Sage.

Wiewelhove, T., Raeder, C., Meyer, T., Kellmann, M., Pfeiffer, M., & Ferrauti, A. (2015). Markers for routine assessment of fatigue and recovery in male and female team sport athletes during high-intensity interval training. *PLoS ONE, 10*(10), e0139801. DOI: 10.1371/journal.pone.0139801

Wiewelhove, T., Raeder, C., Meyer, T., Kellmann, M., Pfeiffer, M., & Ferrauti, A. (2016). Effect of repeated active recovery during a high-intensity shock microcycle on markers of fatigue. *International Journal of Sports Physiology and Performance, 11*, 1060–1066.

Wiewelhove, T., Schneider, C., Schmidt, A., Döweling, A., Meyer, T., Kellmann, M., Pfeiffer, M., & Ferrauti, A. (2018). Active recovery after high-intensity interval-training does not attenuate training adaptation. *Frontiers in Physiology, 9*, 415. DOI: 10.3389/fphys.2018.00415

Williamson, A., & Hoggart, B. (2005). Pain: A review of three commonly used pain rating scales. *Journal of Clinical Nursing, 14*, 798–804.

Zinner, C., Pelka, M., Ferrauti, A., Meyer, T., Pfeiffer, M., & Sperlich, B. (2017). Responses of low and high compression during recovery after repeated sprint training in well trained handball players. *European Journal of Sport Science, 17*, 1304–1310.

Publications using the ARSS and/or the SRSS (Status: December 2018)

Collette, R., Kellmann, M., Ferrauti, A., Meyer, T., & Pfeiffer, M. (2018). Relation between training load and recovery-stress state in high-performance swimming. *Frontiers in Physiology*, *9*, 845. DOI: 10.3389/fphys.2018.00845

Hitzschke, B., Holst, T., Ferrauti, A., Meyer, T., Pfeiffer, M., & Kellmann, M. (2016). Entwicklung des Akutmaßes zur Erfassung von Erholung und Beanspruchung im Sport [Development of the Acute Recovery and Stress Scale]. *Diagnostica*, *62*, 212–226.

Hitzschke, B., Kölling, S., Ferrauti, A., Meyer, T., Pfeiffer, M., & Kellmann, M. (2015). Entwicklung der Kurzskala zur Erfassung von Erholung und Beanspruchung im Sport (KEB) [Development of the Short Recovery and Stress Scale for Sports (SRSS)]. *Zeitschrift für Sportpsychologie*, *22*, 146–161.

Hitzschke, B., Wiewelhove, T., Raeder, C., Ferrauti, A., Meyer, T., Pfeiffer, M., Kellmann, M., & Kölling, S. (2017). Evaluation of psychological measures for the assessment of recovery and stress during a shock-microcycle in strength and high-intensity interval training. *Performance Enhancement & Health*, *5*, 147–157.

Julian, R. A., Meyer, T., Fullagar, H. H. K., Skorski, S., Kellmann, M., Pfeiffer, M., Ferrauti, A., & Hecksteden, A. (2017). Individual patterns in blood-borne indicators of fatigue-trait or chance. *Journal of Strength and Conditioning Research*, *31*, 608–619.

Kölling, S., Hitzschke, B., Holst, T., Ferrauti, A., Meyer, T., Pfeiffer, M., & Kellmann, M. (2015). Validity of the Acute Recovery and Stress Scale: Training monitoring of the German junior national field hockey team. *International Journal of Sports Science & Coaching*, *10*, 529–542.

Kölling, S., Steinacker, J. M., Pfeiffer, M., Ferrauti, A., Meyer, T., & Kellmann, M. (2016). The longer the better: Sleep/wake patterns during preparation of the World Rowing Junior Championships. *Chronobiology International*, *33*, 73–84.

Nässi, A., Ferrauti, A., Meyer, T., Pfeiffer, M., & Kellmann, M. (2017). Development of two short measures for recovery and stress in sport. *European Journal of Sport Science*, *17*, 894–903.

Pelka, M., Ferrauti, A., Meyer, T., Pfeiffer, M., & Kellmann, M. (2017). How does a short, interrupted recovery break affect performance and how is it assessed? A study on acute effects. *International Journal of Sports Physiology and Performance*, *12*(Suppl. 2), S2-114–S2-121.

Pelka, M., Kölling, S., Ferrauti, A., Meyer, T., Pfeiffer, M., & Kellmann, M. (2017). Psychological relaxation between two physical tasks. *Journal of Sports Sciences*, *35*, 216–223.

Pelka, M., Schneider, P., & Kellmann, M. (2018). Development of pre- and post-match morning recovery-stress states during in-season weeks in elite youth football. *Science and Medicine in Football*, *2*, 127–132.

Puta, C., Steidten, T., Baumbach, P., Wöhrl, T., May, R., Kellmann, M., Herbsleb, M., Gabriel, B., Weber, S., Granacher, U., & Gabriel, H. (2018). Standardized assessment of resistance training-induced subjective symptoms and objective signs of immunological stress responses in young athletes. *Frontiers in Physiology*, *9*, 698. DOI: 10.3389/fphys.2018.00698

Puta, C., Weber, S., May, R., Steidten, T., Hildebrandt, P., Gabriel, B., Herbsleb, M., Lesinski, M., Kellmann, M., Granacher, U., & Gabriel, H. (2016). Immun-Score: Entwicklung eines benutzerfreundlichen Instruments zur standarisierten Erfassung von Symptomen für die Differenzierung von belastungsinduzierter und infektbasierter Stressreaktion im Nachwuchsleistungssport [Immune-score: A tool for standardized assessment of symptoms and signs that differentiates immunological stress reactions in youth athletes]. *Leistungssport*, *46*(6), 15–18.

Raeder, C., Wiewelhove, T., de Paula Simola, R. A., Kellmann, M., Meyer, T., Pfeiffer, M., & Ferrauti, A. (2016). Assessment of fatigue and recovery in male and female athletes following six days of intensified strength training. *Journal of Strength and Conditioning Research*, *30*, 3412–3427.

Raeder, C., Wiewelhove, T., Schneider, C., Döweling, A., Kellmann, M., Meyer, T., Pfeiffer, M., & Ferrauti, A. (2017). Effects of active recovery following high-intensity training sessions on muscle function in elite Olympic weightlifters. *Advances in Skeletal Muscle Function Assessment*, *1*(1), 3–12.

Raeder, C., Wiewelhove, T., Westphal-Martinez, M. P., Fernandez-Fernandez, J., de Paula Simola, R. A., Kellmann, M., Meyer, T., Pfeiffer, M., & Ferrauti, A. (2016). Neuromuscular fatigue and physiological responses after five dynamic squat exercise protocols. *Journal of Strength and Conditioning Research*, *30*, 953–965.

Schimpchen, J., Wagner, M., Ferrauti, A., Kellmann, M., Pfeiffer, M., & Meyer, T. (2017). Can cold water immersion enhance recovery in elite Olympic weightlifters?: An individualized perspective. *Journal of Strength and Conditioning Research, 31*, 1569–1576.

Wiewelhove, T., Fernandez-Fernandez, J., Raeder, C., Kappenstein, J., Meyer, T., Kellmann, M., Pfeiffer, M., & Ferrauti, A. (2016). Acute responses and muscle damage in different high-intensity interval running protocols. *Journal of Sports Medicine and Physical Fitness, 56*, 606–615.

Wiewelhove, T., Raeder, C., de Paula Simola, R. A., Schneider, C., Döweling, A., & Ferrauti, A. (2017). Tensiomyographic markers are not sensitive for monitoring muscle fatigue in elite youth athletes: A pilot study. *Frontiers in Physiology, 8*, 406. DOI: 10.3389/fphys.2017.00406

Wiewelhove, T., Raeder, C., Meyer, T., Kellmann, M., Pfeiffer, M., & Ferrauti, A. (2016). Effect of repeated active recovery during a high-intensity shock microcycle on markers of fatigue. *International Journal of Sports Physiology and Performance, 11*, 1060–1066.

Wiewelhove, T., Schneider, C., Döweling, A., Hanakam, F., Meyer, T., Kellmann, M., Pfeiffer, M., & Ferrauti, A. (2018). Effects of different recovery strategies following a half-marathon on fatigue markers in recreational runners. *PLoS ONE, 13*(11), e0207313. DOI: 10.1371/journal.pone.0207313

Wiewelhove, T., Schneider, C., Schmidt, A., Döweling, A., Meyer, T., Kellmann, M., Pfeiffer, M., & Ferrauti, A. (2018). Active recovery after high-intensity interval-training does not attenuate training adaptation. *Frontiers in Physiology, 9*, 415. DOI: 10.3389/fphys.2018.00415

Zinner, C., Pelka, M., Ferrauti, A., Meyer, T., Pfeiffer, M., & Sperlich, B. (2017). Responses of low and high compression during recovery after repeated sprint training in well-trained handball players. *European Journal of Sport Science, 17*, 1304–1310.

Appendix

Appendix overview. Overview of original German adjectives, translated English adjectives, and the final English ARSS after analysis of sample ES1 and ES2.

	Scale	German	English (ES1)	English (ES2)	Final ARSS
Recovery Dimension	Physical Performance Capability (Körperliche Leistungsfähigkeit)	kraftvoll leistungsfähig energiegeladen voller Power	strong energetic physically capable full of power	strong energetic physically capable full of power	strong energetic physically capable full of power
	Mental Performance Capability (Mentale Leistungsfähigkeit)	aufmerksam aufnahmefähig konzentriert mental hellwach	attentive receptive concentrated mentally alert	attentive receptive concentrated mentally alert	attentive receptive concentrated mentally alert
	Emotional Balance (Emotionale Ausgeglichenheit)	zufrieden ausgeglichen gut gelaunt alles im Griff habend	satisfied balanced in a good mood having everything under control	satisfied balanced in a good mood having everything under control stable pleased	in a good mood having everything under control stable pleased
	Overall Recovery (Allgemeiner Erholungszustand)	erholt ausgeruht muskulär locker körperlich entspannt	recovered rested muscle relaxation physically relaxed muscle looseness	recovered rested muscle relaxation physically relaxed	recovered rested muscle relaxation physically relaxed
Stress Dimension	Muscular Stress (Muskuläre Beanspruchung)	muskulär überanstrengt muskulär ermüdet muskulär übersäuert muskulär verhärtet	muscle exhaustion muscle fatigue muscle stiffness muscle soreness muscle tension muscle overstrain	muscle exhaustion muscle fatigue muscle stiffness muscle soreness	muscle exhaustion muscle fatigue muscle stiffness muscle soreness
	Lack of Activation (Aktivierungsmangel)	antriebslos unmotiviert lustlos energielos	unmotivated sluggish unenthusiastic lacking energy	unmotivated sluggish unenthusiastic lacking energy	unmotivated sluggish unenthusiastic lacking energy
	Negative Emotional State (Emotionale Unausgeglichenheit)	bedrückt gestresst genervt leicht reizbar	feeling down short-tempered stressed annoyed	feeling down short-tempered stressed annoyed	feeling down short-tempered stressed annoyed
	Overall Stress (Allgemeiner Beanspruchungszustand)	geschafft entkräftet überlastet körperlich platt	tired worn-out overloaded physically exhausted beat	tired worn-out overloaded physically exhausted	tired worn-out overloaded physically exhausted

Note: ARSS = *Acute Recovery and Stress Scale*; ES = English sample

Appendix ARSS

Appendix ARSS 1 Descriptive data of the ARSS for samples ES1 ($N = 267$).

	M	SD	r_{it}
Physical Performance Capability	*2.77*	*1.05*	
strong	2.98	1.23	.68
energetic	2.57	1.26	.60
physically capable	3.22	1.30	.67
full of power	2.33	1.36	.71
Mental Performance Capability	*2.81*	*0.99*	
attentive	2.86	1.30	.63
receptive	2.64	1.27	.60
mentally alert	2.84	1.25	.62
concentrated	2.91	1.25	.52
Emotional Balance	*2.91*	*0.99*	
satisfied	3.09	1.36	.50
balanced	2.52	1.26	.56
in a good mood	3.28	1.20	.63
having everything under control	2.75	1.37	.53
Overall Recovery	*2.35*	*1.15*	
recovered	2.65	1.46	.61
rested	2.07	1.51	.66
muscle relaxation	2.15	1.36	.64
physically relaxed	2.53	1.40	.63
Muscular Stress	*1.59*	*1.25*	
muscle exhaustion	1.23	1.44	.64
muscle fatigue	1.78	1.52	.76
muscle stiffness	1.65	1.47	.65
muscle soreness	1.71	1.51	.79
Lack of Activation	*1.16*	*1.02*	
unmotivated	0.84	1.26	.59
sluggish	1.46	1.36	.54
unenthusiastic	0.90	1.29	.58
lacking energy	1.45	1.39	.57
Negative Emotional State	*1.02*	*1.05*	
feeling down	0.83	1.25	.61
short-tempered	0.99	1.38	.59
stressed	1.44	1.50	.59
annoyed	0.83	1.23	.64
Overall Stress	*1.52*	*1.18*	
tired	2.17	1.51	.66
worn-out	1.42	1.46	.64
overloaded	1.24	1.34	.65
physically exhausted	1.27	1.43	.73

Note: ARSS = *Acute Recovery and Stress Scale*; ES = English sample

Appendix ARSS 2 Reliability analysis and sample statistics of the original German ARSS scales and items for sample GS3 ($N = 574$).

	Scale	Item	α	M	SD	r_{it}	M	SD
Recovery Dimension	Physical Performance Capability (Körperliche Leistungsfähigkeit)	kraftvoll	.90	3.48	1.27	.77	3.41	1.39
		leistungsfähig				.71	3.97	1.37
		energiegeladen				.79	3.26	1.52
		voller Power				.82	3.29	1.53
	Mental Performance Capability (Mentale Leistungsfähigkeit)	aufmerksam	.84	3.90	1.09	.59	3.99	1.33
		aufnahmefähig				.67	4.19	1.34
		konzentriert				.74	3.93	1.27
		mental hellwach				.68	3.50	1.41
	Emotional Balance (Emotionale Ausgeglichenheit)	zufrieden	.76	3.83	1.09	.55	3.96	1.47
		ausgeglichen				.51	3.52	1.43
		gut gelaunt				.60	4.20	1.37
		alles im Griff habend				.58	3.66	1.42
	Overall Recovery (Allgemeiner Erholungszustand)	erholt	.85	3.07	1.24	.70	3.35	1.44
		ausgeruht				.72	2.97	1.53
		muskulär locker				.65	2.92	1.53
		körperlich entspannt				.70	3.04	1.48
Stress Dimension	Muscular Stress (Muskuläre Beanspruchung)	muskulär überanstrengt	.87	2.27	1.44	.74	2.25	1.60
		muskulär ermüdet				.77	2.56	1.74
		muskulär übersäuert				.75	1.81	1.64
		muskulär verhärtet				.66	2.46	1.76
	Lack of Activation (Aktivierungsmangel)	antriebslos	.86	1.80	1.20	.74	1.59	1.63
		unmotiviert				.70	1.64	1.58
		lustlos				.71	1.63	1.60
		energielos				.65	2.00	1.57
	Negative Emotional State (Emotionale Unausgeglichenheit)	bedrückt	.79	1.94	1.30	.59	1.75	1.67
		gestresst				.56	2.22	1.66
		genervt				.66	1.72	1.56
		leicht reizbar				.61	2.09	1.70
	Overall Stress (Allgemeiner Beanspruchungszustand)	geschafft	.88	2.36	1.42	.71	2.83	1.66
		entkräftet				.76	2.11	1.65
		überlastet				.70	2.03	1.56
		körperlich platt				.76	2.48	1.80

Note: ARSS = *Acute Recovery and Stress Scale*; α = Cronbach's α; r_{it} = corrected item-total correlation; modified from Hitzschke et al. (2016); Means (*M*) and Standard Deviation (*SD*) were added. The original German items are listed since a direct translation of all items is not possible

Appendix ARSS 3 Spearman correlations (r_s) within the ARSS scales for samples GS3 ($N = 574$) and GS5 ($N = 239$).

		Upper data matrix: GS5							
	Scale	PPC	MPC	EB	OR	MS	LA	NES	OS
Recovery Dimension	Physical Performance Capability		**.70**[a]	.40[a]	.63[a]	−.45[a]	−.56[a]	−.23[a]	−.60[a]
	Mental Performance Capability	.69[a]		.46[a]	.48[a]	−.37[a]	−.40[a]	−.21[a]	−.46[a]
	Emotional Balance	.61[a]	.62[a]		.46[a]	−.36[a]	−.41[a]	−.48[a]	−.40[a]
	Overall Recovery	**.71**[a]	.53[a]	.46[a]		−.56[a]	−.46[a]	−.29[a]	−.62[a]
Stress Dimension	Muscular Stress	−.49[a]	−.31[a]	−.21[a]	**−.71**[a]		.49[a]	.32[a]	**.74**[a]
	Lack of Activation	−.68[a]	−.63[a]	−.60[a]	−.47[a]	.38[a]		.51[a]	.52[a]
	Negative Emotional State	−.33[a]	−.40[a]	−.63[a]	−.28[a]	.19[a]	.55[a]		.33[a]
	Overall Stress	**−.71**[a]	−.52[a]	−.44[a]	**−.80**[a]	**.75**[a]	.62[a]	.37[a]	
		Lower data matrix: GS3							

Note: ARSS = *Acute Recovery and Stress Scale*; PPC = *Physical Performance Capability*; MPC = *Mental Performance Capability*; EB = *Emotional Balance*; OR = *Overall Recovery*; MS = *Muscular Stress*; LA = *Lack of Activation*; NES = *Negative Emotional State*; OS = *Overall Stress*; GS = German sample

[a] = $p < .001$; $r \geq .70$ are bolded.

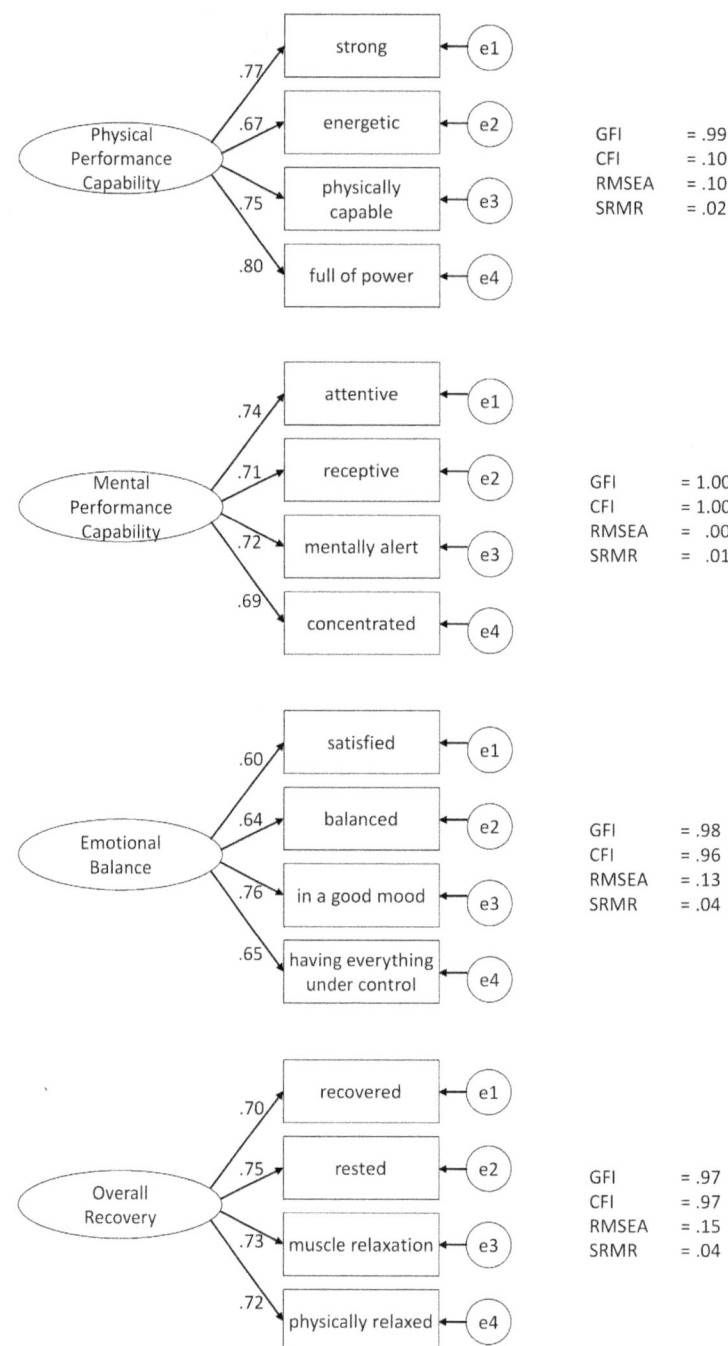

Appendix ARSS 4 Measurement models for the scales of the ARSS as developed by Confirmatory Factor Analysis for ES1.

Note: ARSS = *Acute Recovery and Stress Scale*; ES = English sample; Fit indices data are presented next to the corresponding model. Modified indices are shown in parentheses where error correlations were permitted based on modification indices. GFI = Goodness of Fit Index; CFI = Comparative Fit Index; RMSEA = Root Mean Square Error of Approximation; SRMR = Standardized Root-Mean Square Residual (modified, by permission, from Nässi et al., 2017a, p. 898)

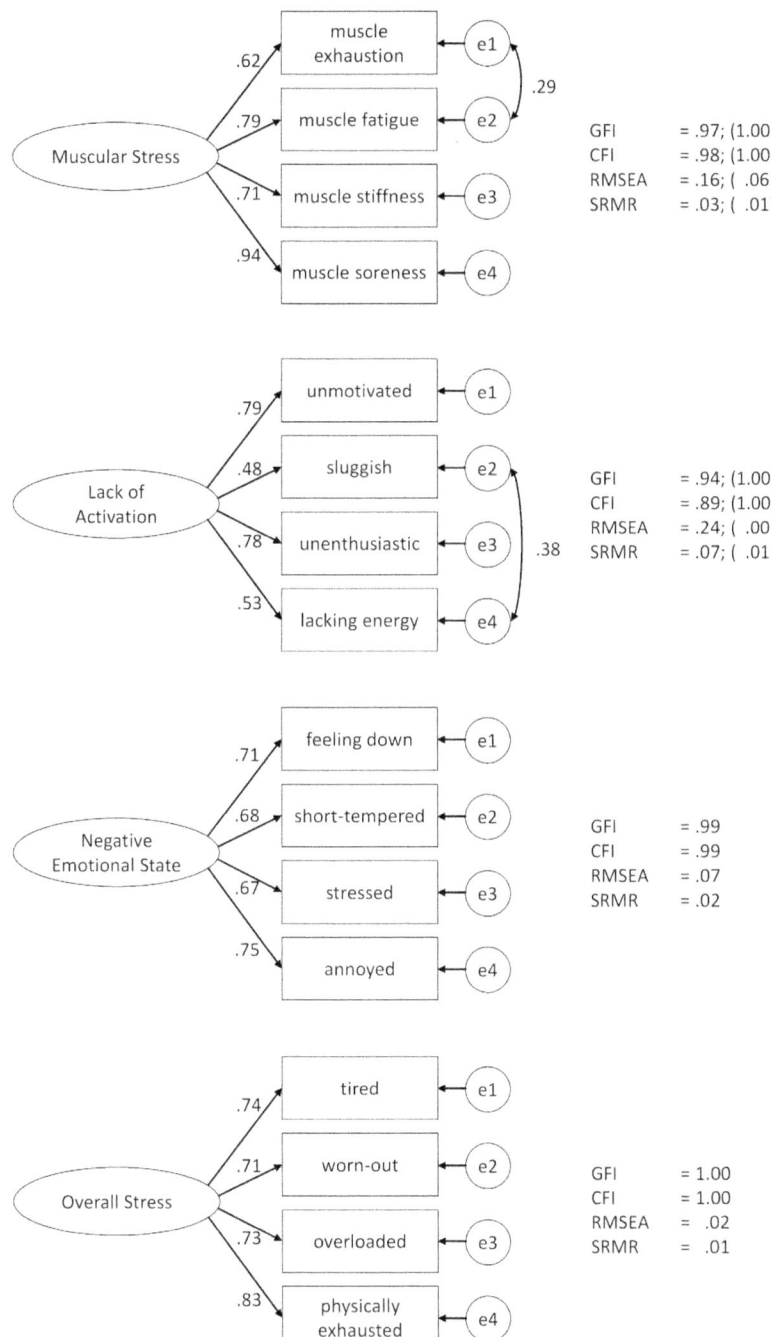

Appendix ARSS 4 (Continued)

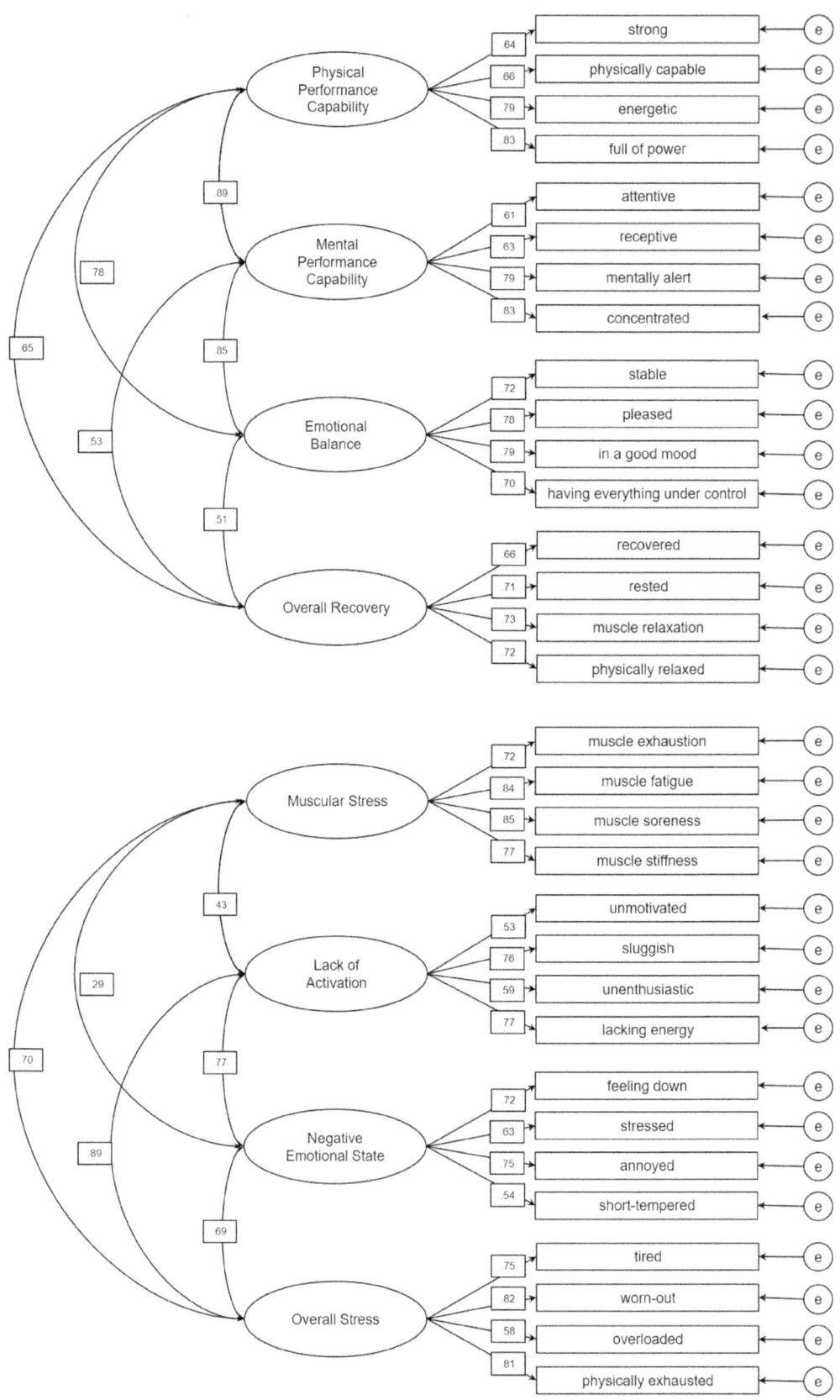

Appendix ARSS 5 Initial measurement model [left] and modified model [right] for the dimensions *Recovery* [top] and *Stress* [bottom] for sample ES2_ANZ (*n* = 379) [for the detailed statistics, see Table 4.9].

Note: ARSS = *Acute Recovery and Stress Scale*; ES = English sample; ANZ = Australia/New Zealand

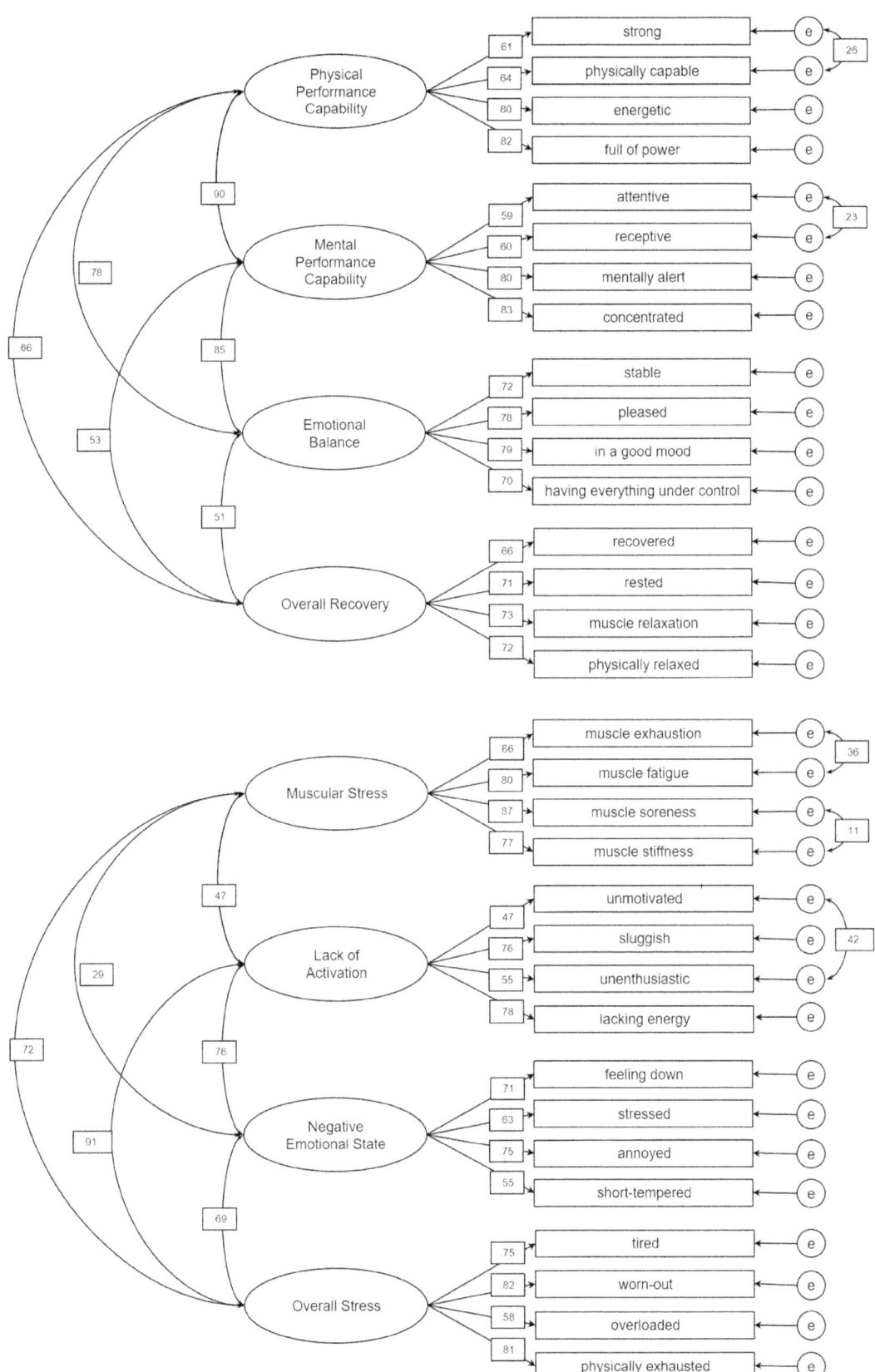

Appendix ARSS 5 (Continued)

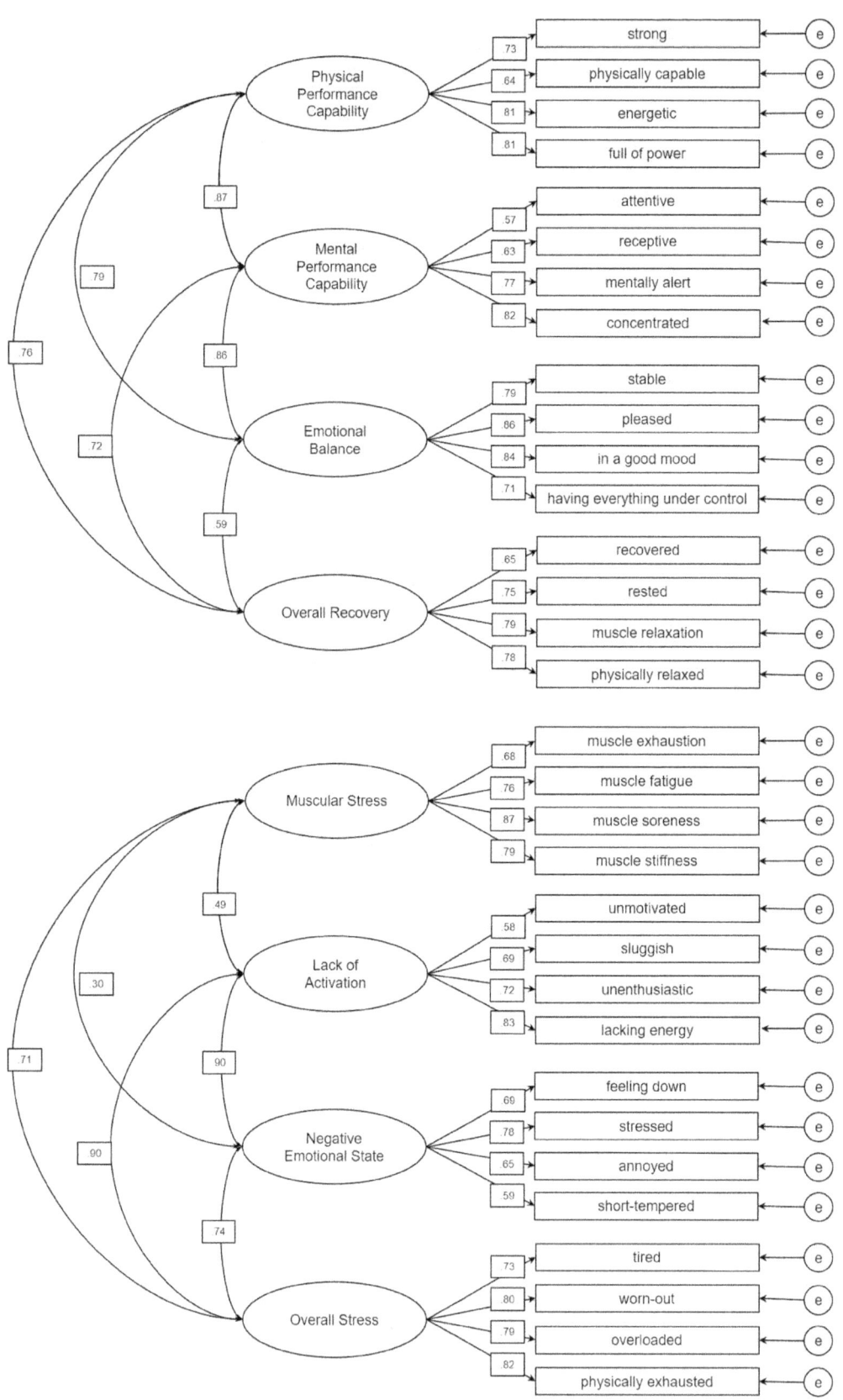

Appendix ARSS 6 Initial measurement model [left] and modified model [right] for the dimensions *Recovery* [top] and *Stress* [bottom] for sample ES2_UK (*n* = 316) [for the detailed statistics, see Table 4.9].

Note: ARSS = *Acute Recovery and Stress Scale*; ES = English sample; UK = United Kingdom

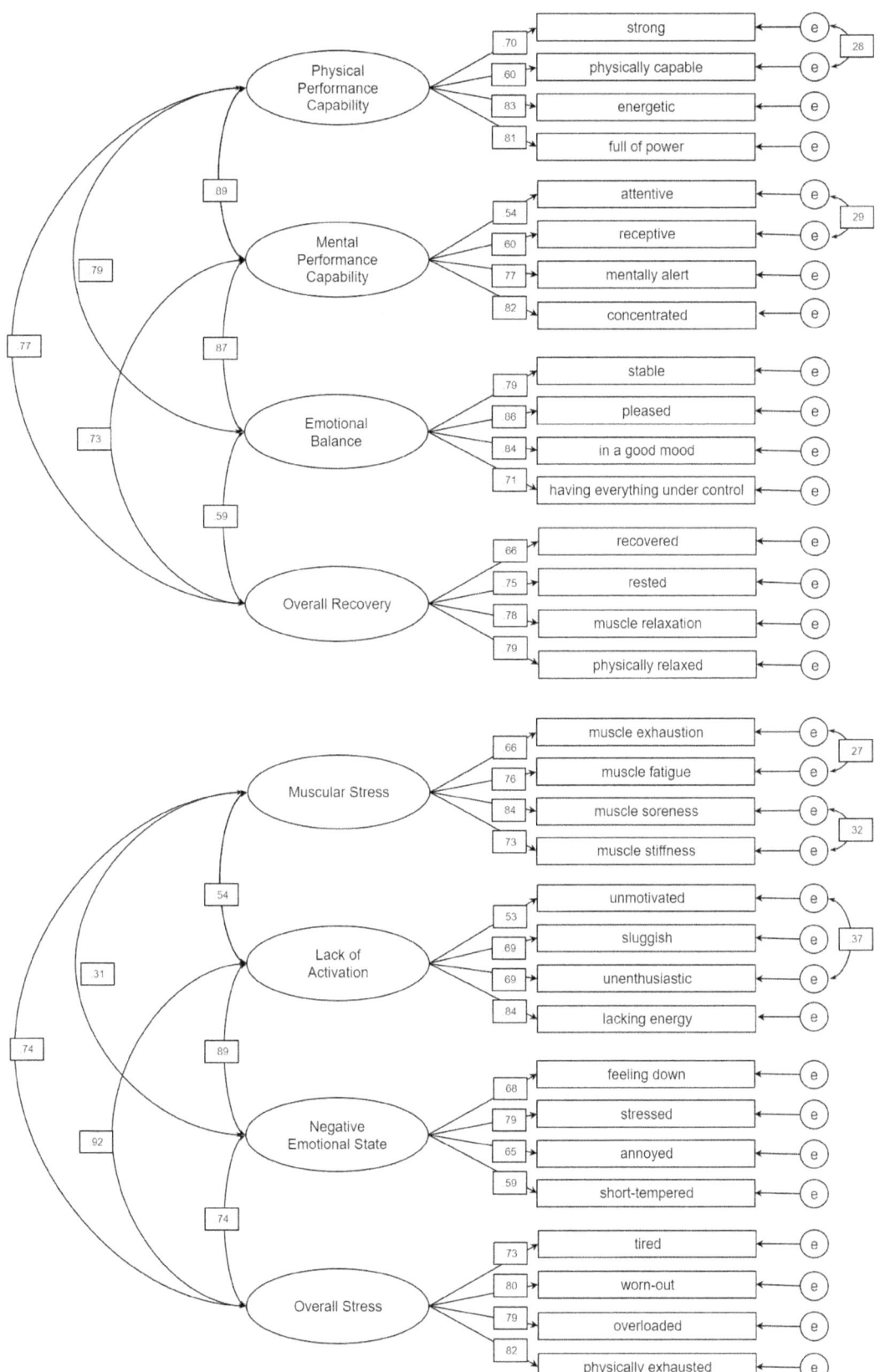

Appendix ARSS 6 (Continued)

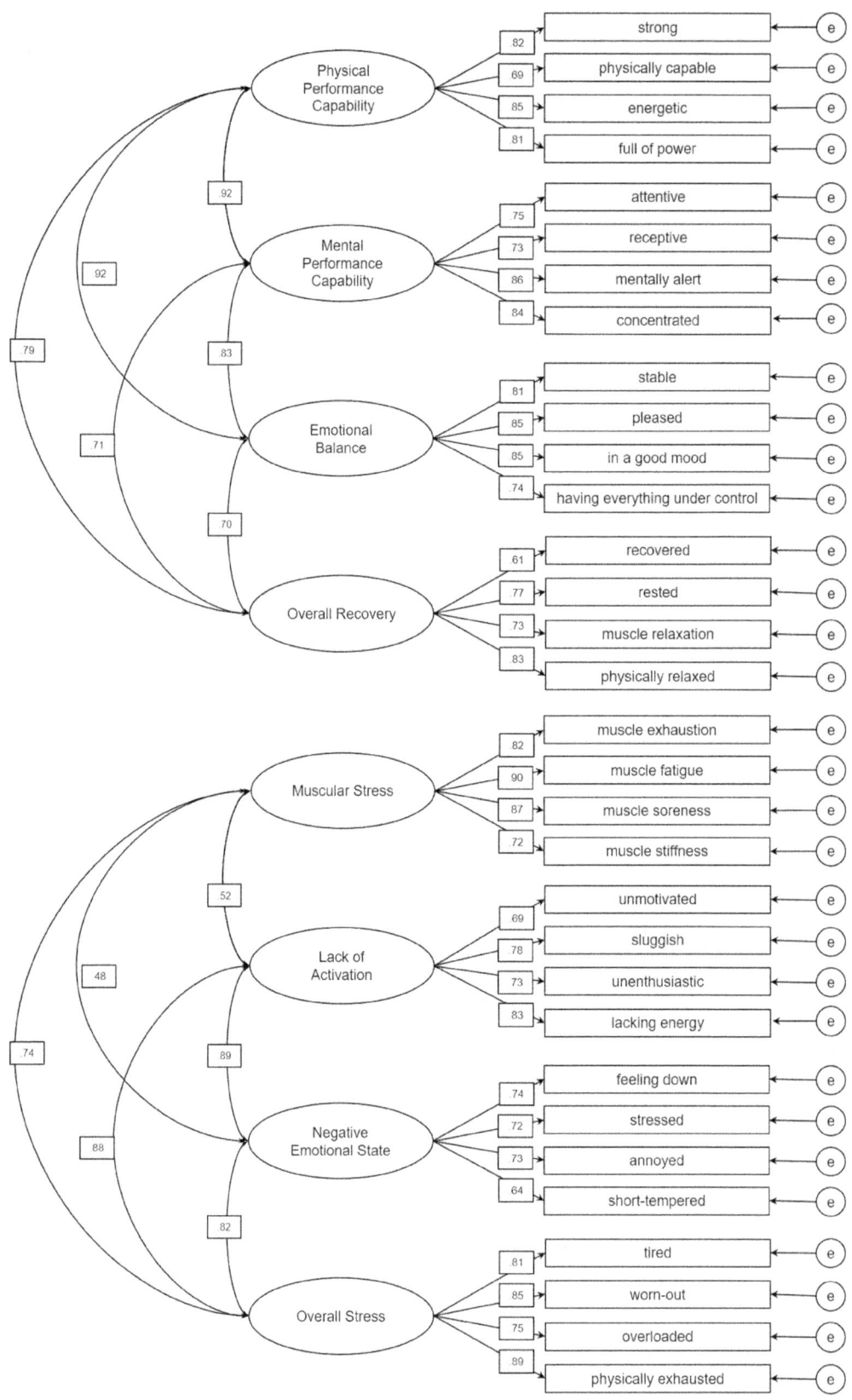

Appendix ARSS 7 Initial measurement model [left] and modified model [right] for the dimensions *Recovery* [top] and *Stress* [bottom] for sample ES2_NA (*n* = 296) [for the detailed statistics, see Table 4.9].

Note: ARSS = *Acute Recovery and Stress Scale*; ES = English sample; NA = North America

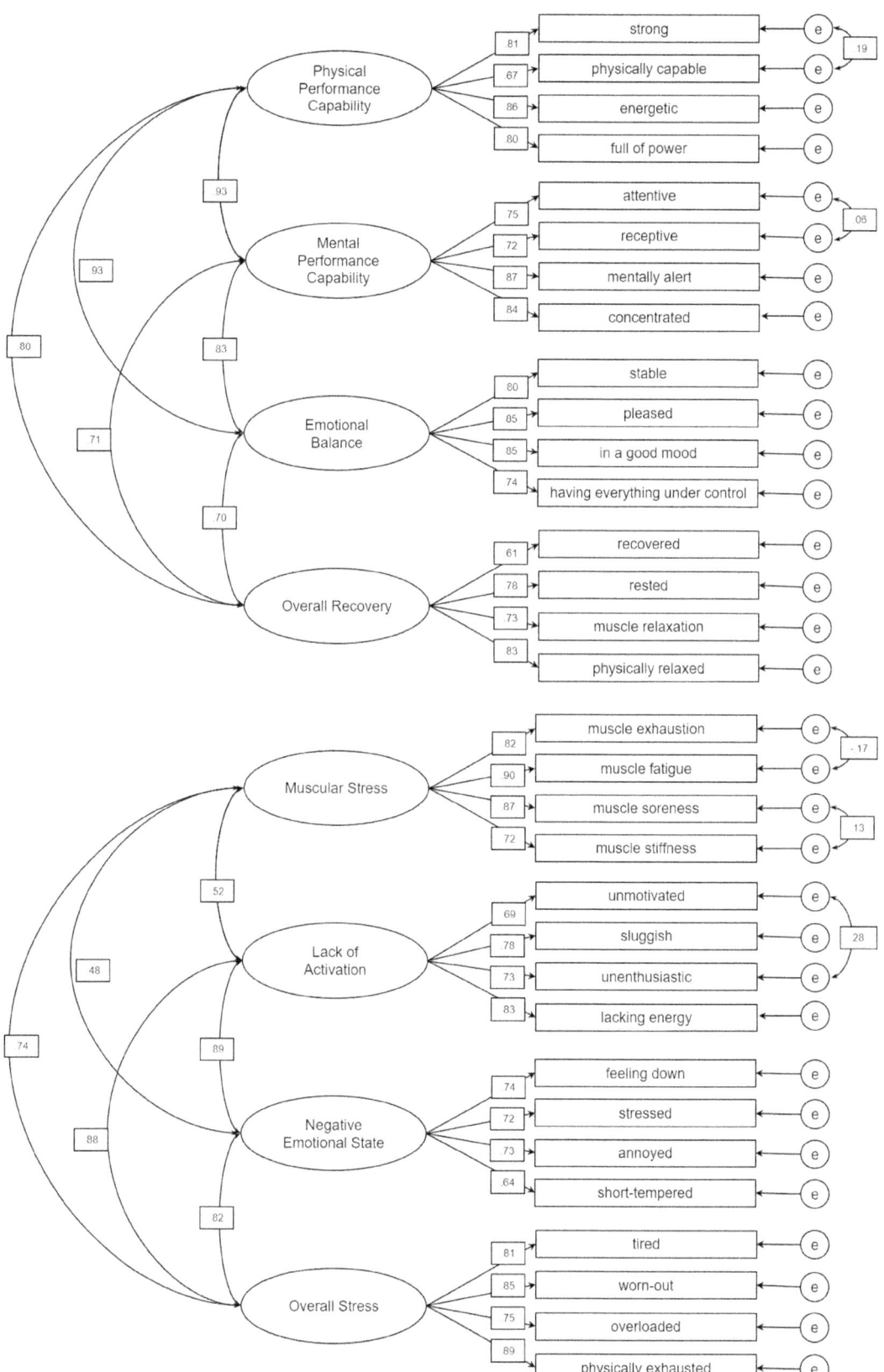

Appendix ARSS 7 (Continued)

Appendix ARSS 8 Correlation of the ARSS scales with the RESTQ-Sport-76 scales for sample GS3 ($N = 574$).

	RESTQ-Sport-76																		
	Overall Stress							Overall Recovery					Sport-specific Stress			Sport-specific Recovery			
	1	2	3	4	5	6	7	8	9	10	11	12	13	14	15	16	17	18	19
PPC	-.43 [a]	-.32 [a]	-.19 [a]	-.23 [a]	-.41 [a]	-.36 [a]	-.55 [a]	.20 [a]	.19 [a]	.68 [a]	.44 [a]	.39 [a]	-.37 [a]	-.44 [a]	-.34 [a]	.68 [a]	.24 [a]	.43 [a]	.45 [a]
MPC	-.44 [a]	-.34 [a]	-.25 [a]	-.24 [a]	-.39 [a]	-.49 [a]	-.44 [a]	.13 [b]	.24 [a]	.53 [a]	.42 [a]	.37 [a]	-.36 [a]	-.42 [a]	-.22 [a]	.55 [a]	.27 [a]	.38 [a]	.44 [a]
EB	-.61 [a]	-.51 [a]	-.34 [a]	-.34 [a]	-.37 [a]	-.42 [a]	-.54 [a]	.22 [a]	.37 [a]	.64 [a]	.65 [a]	.47 [a]	-.39 [a]	-.50 [a]	-.21 [a]	.58 [a]	.31 [a]	.50 [a]	.49 [a]
OR	-.35 [a]	-.23 [a]	-.18 [a]	-.31 [a]	-.46 [a]	-.26 [a]	-.52 [a]	.06 [d]	.13 [b]	.59 [a]	.30 [a]	.36 [a]	-.38 [a]	-.41 [a]	-.42 [a]	.64 [a]	.07 [d]	.21 [a]	.24 [a]
MS	.22 [a]	.17 [a]	.14 [b]	.26 [a]	.35 [a]	.19 [a]	.43 [a]	.06 [d]	-.01 [d]	-.35 [a]	-.12 [a]	-.21 [a]	.37 [a]	.35 [a]	.56 [a]	-.43 [a]	.06 [d]	-.04 [d]	-.06 [d]
LA	.55 [a]	.45 [a]	.31 [a]	.31 [a]	.40 [a]	.46 [a]	.55 [a]	-.14 [b]	-.24 [a]	-.56 [a]	-.42 [a]	-.35 [a]	.42 [a]	.56 [a]	.30 [a]	-.56 [a]	-.25 [a]	-.42 [a]	-.50 [a]
NES	.63 [a]	.64 [a]	.50 [a]	.40 [a]	.31 [a]	.41 [a]	.45 [a]	-.09 [c]	-.34 [a]	-.44 [a]	-.54 [a]	-.38 [a]	.42 [a]	.47 [a]	.17 [a]	-.38 [a]	-.20 [a]	-.33 [a]	-.31 [a]
OS	.42 [a]	.30 [a]	.22 [a]	.31 [a]	.49 [a]	.30 [a]	.59 [a]	-.07 [d]	-.13 [a]	-.55 [a]	-.28 [a]	-.34 [a]	.46 [a]	.48 [a]	.47 [a]	-.60 [a]	-.05 [d]	-.22 [a]	-.25 [a]

Note: [a] = $p < .001$
[b] = $p < .01$
[c] = $p < .05$
[d] = non-significant

Note. ARSS = Acute Recovery and Stress Scale; PPC = Physical Performance Capability; MPC = Mental Performance Capability; EB = Emotional Balance; OR = Overall Recovery; MS = Muscular Stress; LA = Lack of Activation; NES = Negative Emotional State; OS = Overall Stress; RESTQ-Sport-76 = Recovery-Stress Questionnaire for Athletes; RESTQ-Sport-76 scales: 1 = General Stress; 2 = Emotional Stress; 3 = Social Stress; 4 = Conflicts/Pressure; 5 = Fatigue; 6 = Lack of Energy; 7 = Physical Complaints; 8 = Success; 9 = Social Recovery; 10 = Physical Recovery; 11 = General Well-being; 12 = Sleep Quality; 13 = Disturbed Breaks; 14 = Emotional Exhaustion; 15 = Injury; 16 = Being in Shape; 17 = Personal Accomplishment; 18 = Self-Efficacy; 19 = Self-Regulation

Appendix SRSS

Appendix SRSS 1 Descriptive data of the SRSS for sample ES1 ($n = 254$).

		M	SD	r_{it}
Short Recovery Scale	Physical Performance Capability	2.86	1.31	.59
	Mental Performance Capability	3.04	1.18	.65
	Emotional Balance	2.99	1.29	.50
	Overall Recovery	2.47	1.24	.59
Short Stress Scale	Muscular Stress	1.71	1.35	.30
	Lack of Activation	1.28	1.28	.61
	Negative Emotional State	1.02	1.29	.52
	Overall Stress	1.45	1.35	.72

Note: SRSS = *Short Recovery and Stress Scale*; ES = English sample.

Appendix SRSS 2 Reliability analysis, sample statistics and Spearman correlations (r_s) of the SRSS in study GS3 ($N = 574$).

	Item	α	M	SD	r_{it}	PPC	MPC	EB	OR	MS	LA	NES
Short Recovery Scale	Physical Performance Capability	.70	4.17	1.47	.62							
	Mental Performance Capability		4.42	1.30	.51	.52 [a]						
	Emotional Balance		4.28	1.48	.37	.33 [a]	.31 [a]					
	Overall Recovery		3.74	1.58	.53	.59 [a]	.38 [a]	.29 [a]				
Short Stress Scale	Muscular Stress	.76	3.06	1.83	.49	−.32 [a]	−.22 [a]	−.07 [a]	−.45 [a]			
	Lack of Activation		2.42	1.85	.58	−.33 [a]	−.37 [a]	−.28 [a]	−.26 [a]	.33 [a]		
	Negative Emotional State		2.35	1.85	.48	−.15 [a]	−.26 [a]	−.37 [a]	−.17 [a]	.24 [a]	.55 [a]	
	Overall Stress		2.93	1.84	.66	−.39 [a]	−.32 [a]	−.15 [a]	−.49 [a]	.62 [a]	.51 [a]	.40 [a]

Note: SRSS = *Short Recovery and Stress Scale*; PPC = *Physical Performance Capability*; MPC = *Mental Performance Capability*; EB = *Emotional Balance*; OR = *Overall Recovery*; MS = *Muscular Stress*; LA = *Lack of Activation*; NES = *Negative Emotional State*; GS = German sample; α = Cronbach's α; r_{it} = corrected item-total correlation

[a] = $p < .001$; modified from Hitzschke et al. (2016)

Appendix SRSS 3 Spearman correlations (r_s) of the SRSS with the RESTQ-Sport-76 in study GS3 ($N = 574$).

	RESTQ–Sport–76																		
	Overall Stress							Overall Recovery					Sport–specific Stress			Sport–specific Recovery			
	1	2	3	4	5	6	7	8	9	10	11	12	13	14	15	16	17	18	19
PPC	-.29	-.19	-.12	-.17	-.31	-.22	-.42	.10	.07	.46	.27	.24	-.21	-.30	-.28	.46	.13	.24	.25
MPC	-.32	-.23	-.16	-.14	-.29	-.26	-.31	.08	.10	.37	.26	.31	-.25	-.31	-.19	.36	.16	.22	.29
EB	-.30	-.39	-.25	-.26	-.25	-.20	-.30	.07	.24	.37	.44	.28	-.26	-.29	-.13	.32	.19	.29	.30
OR	-.30	-.19	-.17	-.25	-.37	-.17	-.40	.08	.06	.45	.21	.24	-.35	-.35	-.36	.42	.03	.18	.21
MS	.23	.17	.18	.23	.33	.24	.38	.02	-.06	-.35	-.13	-.18	.29	.31	.45	-.40	-.02	-.11	-.12
LA	.49	.39	.29	.26	.32	.48	.43	-.13	-.25	-.47	-.39	-.31	.34	.42	.18	-.45	-.18	-.38	-.48
NES	.58	.60	.45	.38	.28	.46	.39	-.07	-.29	-.43	-.48	-.30	.35	.41	.15	-.37	-.20	-.34	-.31
OS	.37	.28	.23	.28	.43	.34	.47	-.10	-.15	-.48	-.25	-.26	.44	.40	.35	-.53	-.10	-.22	-.27

Note: All correlations were significant $p < .001$; GS = German sample; SRSS = Short Recovery and Stress Scale; PPC = Physical Performance Capability; MPC = Mental Performance Capability; EB = Emotional Balance; OR = Overall Recovery; MS = Muscular Stress; LA = Lack of Activation; NES = Negative Emotional State; OS = Overall Stress; RESTQ-Sport-76 = Recovery-Stress Questionnaire for Athletes; RESTQ-Sport-76 scales: 1 = General Stress; 2 = Emotional Stress; 3 = Social Stress; 4 = Conflicts/Pressure; 5 = Fatigue; 6 = Lack of Energy; 7 = Physical Complaints; 8 = Success; 9 = Social Recovery; 10 = Physical Recovery; 11 = General Well-being; 12 = Sleep Quality; 13 = Disturbed Breaks; 14 = Emotional Exhaustion; 15 = Injury; 16 = Being in Shape; 17 = Personal Accomplishment; 18 = Self-Efficacy; 19 = Self-Regulation

Name/Code Date/Time

Acute Recovery and Stress Scale

Below there is a list of expressions that describe different states of recovery and stress. Please rate each item and mark the number that most closely applies to you **right now**.

At the moment I feel / I am …	does not apply at all						fully applies
1 recovered	0	1	2	3	4	5	6
2 muscle exhaustion	0	1	2	3	4	5	6
3 pleased	0	1	2	3	4	5	6
4 unmotivated	0	1	2	3	4	5	6
5 attentive	0	1	2	3	4	5	6
6 feeling down	0	1	2	3	4	5	6
7 strong	0	1	2	3	4	5	6
8 tired	0	1	2	3	4	5	6
9 rested	0	1	2	3	4	5	6
10 muscle fatigue	0	1	2	3	4	5	6
11 stable	0	1	2	3	4	5	6
12 sluggish	0	1	2	3	4	5	6
13 receptive	0	1	2	3	4	5	6
14 stressed	0	1	2	3	4	5	6
15 physically capable	0	1	2	3	4	5	6
16 worn-out	0	1	2	3	4	5	6
17 muscle relaxation	0	1	2	3	4	5	6
18 unenthusiastic	0	1	2	3	4	5	6
19 in a good mood	0	1	2	3	4	5	6
20 annoyed	0	1	2	3	4	5	6
21 mentally alert	0	1	2	3	4	5	6
22 muscle soreness	0	1	2	3	4	5	6
23 energetic	0	1	2	3	4	5	6
24 overloaded	0	1	2	3	4	5	6
25 physically relaxed	0	1	2	3	4	5	6
26 muscle stiffness	0	1	2	3	4	5	6
27 having everything under control	0	1	2	3	4	5	6
28 lacking energy	0	1	2	3	4	5	6
29 concentrated	0	1	2	3	4	5	6
30 short-tempered	0	1	2	3	4	5	6
31 full of power	0	1	2	3	4	5	6
32 physically exhausted	0	1	2	3	4	5	6

© Kellmann & Kölling (2019)

Name/Code Date/Time

Scoring key of the ARSS

Recovery Dimension				Stress Dimension			
1 Physical Performance Capability	*2* Mental Performance Capability	*3* Emotional Balance	*4* Overall Recovery	*5* Muscular Stress	*6* Lack of Activation	*7* Negative Emotional State	*8* Overall Stress
7	5	3	1	2	4	6	8
15	13	11	9	10	12	14	16
23	21	19	17	22	18	20	24
31	29	27	25	26	28	30	32
Sum	Sum	Sum	Sum	Sum	Sum	Sum	Sum
Mean	Mean	Mean	Mean	Mean	Mean	Mean	Mean

© Kellmann & Kölling (2019)

| Name/Code | Date/Time |

Scoring Profile of the
Acute Recovery and Stress Scale

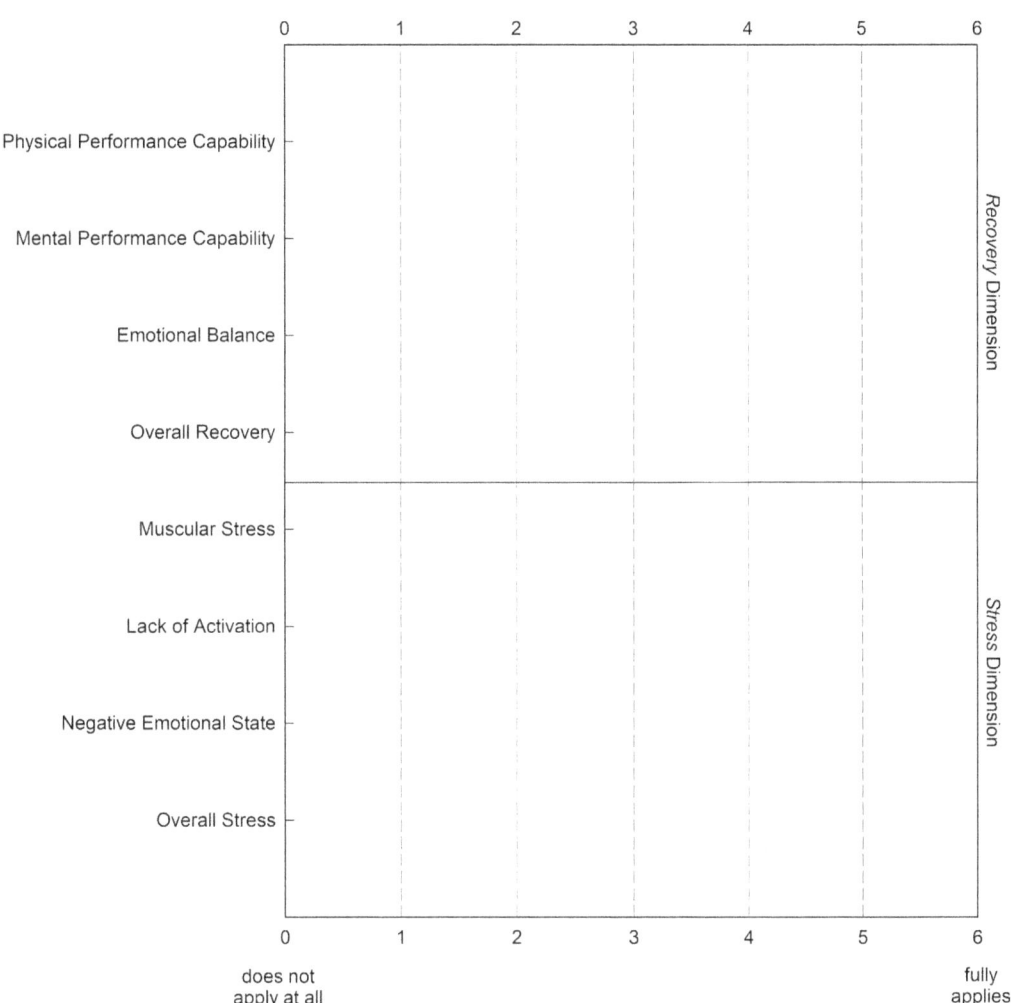

© Kellmann & Kölling (2019)

Name/Code Date/Time

Short Recovery Scale

Below you find a list of expressions that describe different aspects of your current state of recovery. Rate how you feel **right now** in relation to your best ever recovery state.

Physical Performance Capability

e.g
strong,
physically capable,
energetic,
full of power

does not apply at all 0 — 1 — 2 — 3 — 4 — 5 — 6 fully applies

---

Mental Performance Capability

e.g
attentive,
receptive,
mentally alert,
concentrated

does not apply at all 0 — 1 — 2 — 3 — 4 — 5 — 6 fully applies

---

Emotional Balance

e.g
pleased,
stable,
in a good mood,
having everything under control

does not apply at all 0 — 1 — 2 — 3 — 4 — 5 — 6 fully applies

---

Overall Recovery

e.g
recovered,
rested,
muscle relaxation,
physically relaxed

does not apply at all 0 — 1 — 2 — 3 — 4 — 5 — 6 fully applies

---

© Kellmann & Kölling (2019)

| Name/Code | Date/Time |

Short Stress Scale

Below you find a list of expressions that describe different aspects of your current state of stress. Rate how you feel **right now** in relation to your highest ever stress state.

Muscular Stress
e.g.
muscle exhaustion,
muscle fatigue,
muscle soreness,
muscle stiffness

does not apply at all 0 — 1 — 2 — 3 — 4 — 5 — 6 fully applies

---

Lack of Activation
e.g.
unmotivated,
sluggish,
unenthusiastic,
lacking energy

does not apply at all 0 — 1 — 2 — 3 — 4 — 5 — 6 fully applies

---

Negative Emotional State
e.g.
feeling down,
stressed,
annoyed,
short-tempered

does not apply at all 0 — 1 — 2 — 3 — 4 — 5 — 6 fully applies

---

Overall Stress
e.g.
tired,
worn-out,
overloaded,
physically exhausted

does not apply at all 0 — 1 — 2 — 3 — 4 — 5 — 6 fully applies

---

© Kellmann & Kölling (2019)

Name/Code	Date/Time

Short Recovery Scale | Short Stress Scale

Below you find a list of expressions that describe different aspects of your current state of recovery. Rate how you feel **right now** in relation to your best ever recovery state.

Below you find a list of expressions that describe different aspects of your current state of stress. Rate how you feel **right now** in relation to your highest ever stress state.

Physical Performance Capability
e.g strong, physically capable, energetic, full of power

does not apply at all 0 — 1 — 2 — 3 — 4 — 5 — 6 fully applies

Muscular Stress
e.g muscle exhaustion, muscle fatigue, muscle soreness, muscle stiffness

does not apply at all 0 — 1 — 2 — 3 — 4 — 5 — 6 fully applies

Mental Performance Capability
e.g attentive, receptive, mentally alert concentrated

does not apply at all 0 — 1 — 2 — 3 — 4 — 5 — 6 fully applies

Lack of Activation
e.g unmotivated, sluggish, unenthusiastic, lacking energy

does not apply at all 0 — 1 — 2 — 3 — 4 — 5 — 6 fully applies

Emotional Balance
e.g pleased, stable, in a good mood, having everything under control

does not apply at all 0 — 1 — 2 — 3 — 4 — 5 — 6 fully applies

Negative Emotional State
e.g feeling down, stressed, annoyed, short-tempered

does not apply at all 0 — 1 — 2 — 3 — 4 — 5 — 6 fully applies

Overall Recovery
e.g recovered, rested, muscle relaxation, physically relaxed

does not apply at all 0 — 1 — 2 — 3 — 4 — 5 — 6 fully applies

Overall Stress
e.g tired, worn-out, overloaded, physically exhausted

does not apply at all 0 — 1 — 2 — 3 — 4 — 5 — 6 fully applies

© Kellmann & Kölling (2019)

| Name/Code | Date/Time |

Scoring Profile of the Short Recovery and Stress Scale

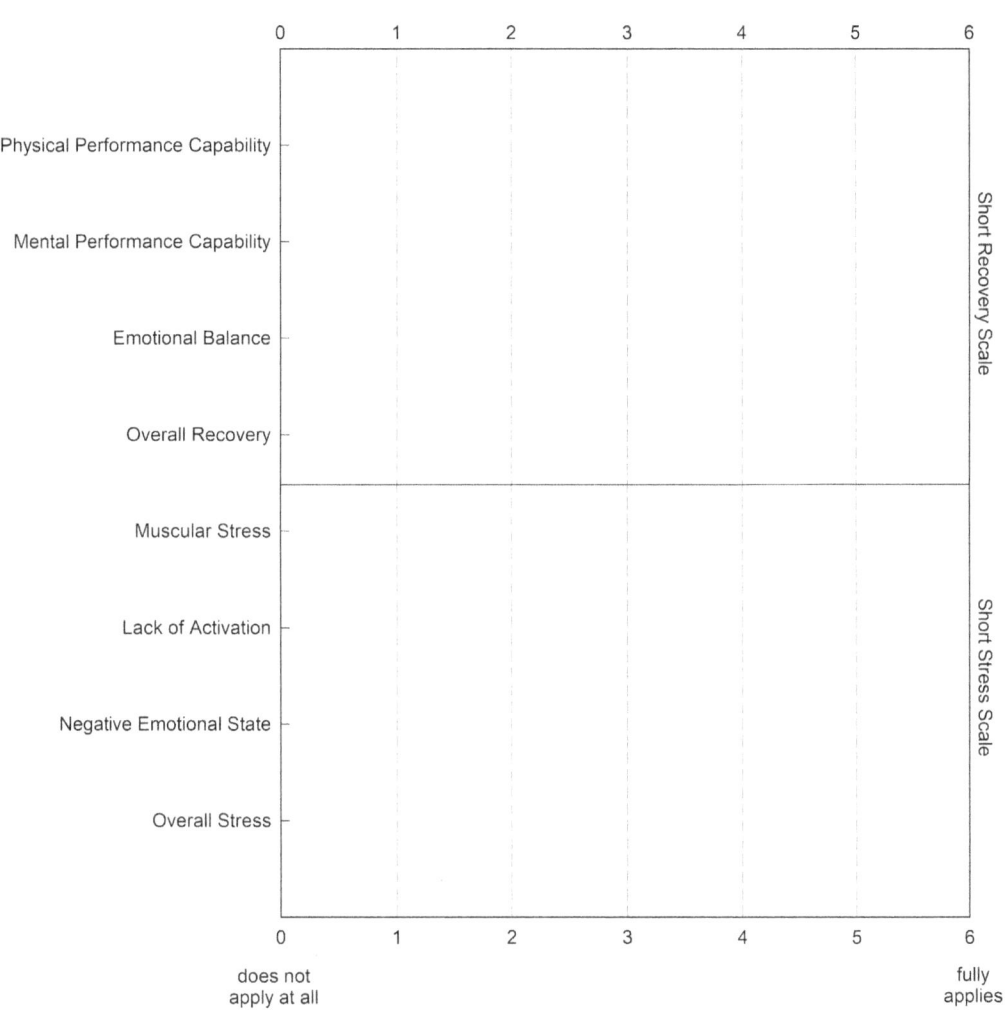

© Kellmann & Kölling (2019)

About the authors

Michael Kellmann

Prof. Michael Kellmann, Head of Unit of Sport Psychology at the Faculty of Sport Science, Ruhr University Bochum (Germany) and Honorary Professor at the School of Human Movement and Nutrition Sciences, The University of Queensland (Australia), is a member of several psychological associations and societies. His current research activities include overtraining prevention and recovery enhancement, regeneration management in elite sports, sport-psychological diagnostics and intervention, as well as the development of research tools for the assessment of recovery. He successfully applied for several millions of euros in total for third-party research grants and applied consulting projects. He has (co-)authored numerous books and articles concerning regeneration and recovery in elite athletes. Michael has consulted with and conducted research for individual athletes, professional sport clubs, and organizations in several countries and different types of sport.

Sarah Kölling

Dr. Sarah Kölling is a Senior Researcher in Sport Psychology at the Faculty of Sport Science at Ruhr University Bochum (Germany). While creating this manual, she was also holding a post-doc position at Stellenbosch University (South Africa). She completed her dissertation within the research project '*Optimization of Training and Competition: Management of Regeneration in Elite Sports* (REGman)' and acquired profound knowledge within sleep research in applied settings (e.g., jet lag). Sarah also examined the effectiveness of recovery strategies in laboratory as well as field studies (e.g., power napping). She was involved in the development process of the ARSS and SRSS as well as its application in several monitoring studies. Currently, she works on the transferability and application of the ARSS/SRSS in non-sport settings.

Index

adaptation 16, 18, 34, 39, 41, 53, 64
application 1, 3, 8, 16, 39, 58, **62**
assessment 2, 5, 16–19, 40–42, 58–**62**

baseline 17, 34, 41, 51, 55, 60
Borg's Rating of Perceived Exhaustion (RPE) 4, 5

case studies 63
Classical Test Theory 14, 15, 19
comparison of ARSS and SRSS 56
competition 2–5, 17, 19, 34, 41, 42, **62**
Confirmatory Factor Analyses (CFA) 1, 7–9, 24–28, 40
creatine kinase 5, 34, 53, 59
Cronbach's α 1, 8, 9, 19, 21, 28, 38, 42, 43, 55
cultural background x, 8

Delayed-Onset Muscle Soreness (DOMS) 4–13, 28–32, 45–49, 55–**62**
dose-response relationship 34, 55
duration 1, 16, 40, 43, 44, 61

evaluation 3, 14, 17, 40, 41, 58
Exploratory Factor Analyses 6, 14, 24
exploratory model development 6, 7

granulocytes 37

homogeneity 14, 19, 24, 42, 43, 58

immunological responses 34, 38
instruction 4, 16, 38, 40, 55
internal consistency 1, 19, 42, 43

language x, xi, 9, 14, 19, 24–28, 38, 42, 46, 49, 55
load 2–5, 7, 17, 34, 35, 41, 55
lymphocytes 37

maladaptation 2
methods of analysis 14
monitoring x, 1, 3–9, 16–17, 34, 39, 41, 51, 55, 58, 60, **62**
mood 4, 18, 22, 28–32, 44–50

Overreaching: functional 2, non-functional 2, 3
overtraining syndrome 2–4

performance i, 2–5, 16, 34, 39, 40, 53, 58, **62**
physiological response 34, 53
preparatory phase 6, 7
Profile of Mood States (POMS) 4, 5, 9, 12, 14, 28–32, 45–50, 57
psychometrics x

rating scale 38, 55
Recovery: definition 2, insufficient 2, 3
Recovery-Stress Questionnaire for Athletes (RESTQ-Sport) 5–14, 28–32, 38, 45–48, 55, 57–**62**
recovery-stress state i, x, 3, 5, 16, 19, 31, 34, 38, 39, 42, 44, 45, 49, 55, 56, 60–62
reference values 19, 42
regeneration 2, 3, 14, 16, 18, 22, 40, 41, 63
reliability xi, 1, 10, 12, 19, 21, 24, 42, 44, **61**

samples 10–14
scope 16, 39
sensitivity to change 1, 9, 13, 31–33, 49, 50, 55, 58, 62
Session-RPE 4, 35
Short Recovery Scale 1, 8, 39–58
Short Stress Scale 1, 8, 39–58
South Africa **12**, 14
sport-scientific practice 16, 39
sport-scientific research 16, 39
studies: field xi, 6, 7, 32, 49, 51, laboratory 6, 7, 31, 40, 49

test development 6
tool i, x, 3–5, 17, 18, 39, 41, 56–62

underrecovery syndrome 3
usage in practice 60

validity 22–38, 44–55

For Product Safety Concerns and Information please contact our EU representative GPSR@taylorandfrancis.com
Taylor & Francis Verlag GmbH, Kaufingerstraße 24, 80331 München, Germany

www.ingramcontent.com/pod-product-compliance
Lightning Source LLC
Chambersburg PA
CBHW081148230426
43664CB00018B/2852